Healthy Living
Doesn't Have to
SUCK

GUIDED COACHING WORKBOOK:
Lasting Positive Habit Change is Within Your Reach!

Melyssa Allen, MA, CHWC, DipACLM

Healthy Living Doesn't Have to SUCK

Cover design by Evelyn Aguilar of HeyEve
Photo by Alicia Ifill of Alicia Ifill Photography
Editing by Mar Dolan of Spark Editorial Agency

ISBN: 979-8-218-10406-1

For more information, visit
https://healthylivingdoesnthavetosuck.com
www.melyssawithawhy.com
or email info@melyssawithawhy.com

Dedication

For my incredibly loving, supportive parents, Bobby & Susan Allen, who have always believed in their little girl achieving her wildest dreams.

For Matt, who continuously puts up with my shenanigans and loves me in all my chaos!

For Buddy, the most amazing soul dog I could have ever asked for, my forced emotional support animal, and my greatest heartbreak waiting to happen - I love you furrrever.

TABLE OF CONTENTS

PREFACE

Hey y'all, my name is Melyssa with a WHY and I want to start by extending my sincerest gratitude that you have this book in your hands right now! I can't tell you how many times I almost talked myself out of not following through with writing this book, because I didn't feel worthy of writing a book about lifestyle change. I am hopeful that you will enjoy this journey together and it will lead you to a new way of approaching behavior changes that stick!

And listen y'all–this book in your hands is called a **work**book for a reason...because you've gotta do the **WORK!** So grab a pen and a journal to keep track of your answers for the reflection prompts as we go. You can also download some freebies at **healthylivingdoesnthavetosuck.com/bonus** to go along with the content! You won't experience healthy lifestyle changes if you're not willing to put in some effort, try out new things, or throw in the towel and quit at your first little hiccup along the way. That's not how we roll anymore–and I say "WE" throughout this book quite often, because I want you to know that I am in this with you too. We are on the same team as we work toward building our positive health habits together!

Now–if you're looking for a completely comprehensive overview of the research on healthy lifestyle habits–*this ain't it!* While I do touch on some of the research, you won't be finding an exhaustive literature review here. You know what else you won't be finding in this book?

Perfection. There are bound to be typos, grammatical errors, times where I may accidentally repeat myself, and the flow of the book might not be its best yet. My hope is that these imperfections won't deter you from the book, but rather that it teaches you to embrace the idea that imperfect action can still lead to massive impact. Especially when it comes to a behavior change journey, we can get so fixated on trying to do everything perfectly, that it ultimately leads to us getting in our own way! Let's agree to cut out that "striving for perfection" shit–OK?

Oops–I should probably mention that while I didn't end up curse like a sailor throughout this book, there are definitely some expletives along the way. If reading a book with "sentence enhancers" isn't your thing, then you might want to find another book to read. Still with me? AWESOME–but don't say I didn't warn you and then come after me in the book reviews and comments!

If you are reading this page right now, that means you have the original version of this book–the one I released when I REALLY didn't feel ready to, but I did it anyway. That being said, if you do have any suggestions or constructive feedback for me along the way, I would love for you to share it with me! My contact information is at the end of the book, and I would genuinely appreciate hearing from you!

I wrote this book to be conversational, so it's like I'm right there with you as your coach! While the coaching process is a two-way interaction, I did my best to provide guided prompts and reflections for your self-guided coaching experience. My focus for this book is providing information to help increase your confidence, boost your motivation, and provide you with tangible tips for swapping out behaviors that pull you away from your healthiest, happiest self with behaviors that push you closer toward that healthiest, happiest version of YOU! Does that include every healthy living trick in the book? Absolutely not! I do intend to share what has worked well for me, what is supported by research, and ask you some powerful questions so you can begin brainstorming your own strategies for success!

WOW! Oh my gosh, OK–should we get started now?! YAAAY!
I am so excited to be here with you as you begin building positive habits *for life!*

Let's get to it y'all–get ready to start your Healthy Living Doesn't Have to SUCK journey!

INTRODUCTION

*"Don't be ashamed of your story;
it will inspire others."*
-Anonymous

Hey, Change Makers! That's right, from this point on I want you to think of yourself as someone making positive changes in your life–because that's why this book is in your hands, right?! You want to learn how to let go of the struggle, build a plan for success, and figure out how to pick yourself back up after the setbacks you've encountered. Just acknowledging that there is an area of your life that you want to enhance is exciting! As you go through this book, you will build your positive lifestyle "toolbox" to begin creating your happiest, healthiest life!

As you're starting this workbook, you might think, *Great, another person's ridiculous success story that I'll end up unconsciously comparing myself to...* I can tell you, that's not what I want for you. In fact, that's what makes this book different.

You will NOT be hearing about my tremendous and successful lifestyle transformation. Right now, I am on the verge of being diagnosed with high cholesterol and can't fit into any of my pants besides the stretchy leggings. I'm also struggling to fight the same habits I've worked so hard to undo years ago. Moreover, I am currently recovering from a massive setback in my mental and emotional well-being *(ahem, thanks COVID pandemic...).* This book will not be a "just do what I did" self-help manual telling you how I've got my life all figured out and how I'm my happiest and healthiest self. I hope that doesn't scare you off from going through this book because, ultimately, my hope is for us to work through this wild ride to better health *together.*

HOW THIS BOOK CAN HELP YOU

I want to make it perfectly clear that I am not going to be asking you to restrict or deprive yourself of anything, such as carbs, soda, meat, sugar, etc. While I may encourage you to reduce your intake of some of these things, I won't tell you to quit ANYTHING cold turkey! Making drastic changes like that can be pretty miserable, and this book is entitled *Healthy Living Doesn't Have to SUCK* for a reason. So instead, what you can expect to learn more about is what promotes health. I will also discuss the behaviors that put our health at risk, how to recognize where you are starting RIGHT NOW, and how to begin small habit changes. Making those smaller changes will help you create positive momentum in your life and ultimately build into a larger lifestyle transformation!

Why is this important to know? Well, if you are anything like me, you know how difficult it is to stay motivated. I have started and quit more fitness and nutrition programs than I care to count...The problem I kept running into was trying to follow every guideline of the program and using my willpower to avoid my guilty pleasures...

Since you are reading this book right now, I'm guessing that you probably feel like you've tried everything out there to lose weight, build healthier habits, or get some control over your life. You might have even gone "all in" after thinking you've finally had enough and had hit your rock bottom...but instead of digging yourself out, you got hit with the old "but wait, there's more!"

Perhaps, what you once believed was a final straw fueled your desperate desire to finally change. However, that desperation only led to a brief spurt of motivation and dedication before you fell down the dark, unfortunate spiral of self-sabotage yet again…

OUCH…! That gets me every time because I've lived that cycle more times than I'd like to admit…!

Why is it SO freaking hard to change our behaviors?! UGH! I swear, no matter how many degrees or certifications I get, I sometimes still feel stuck. And that's why I wanted to write this book… because I can sympathize with how you might have felt or may be feeling right now:

Stuck.
Unhealthy.
Fat.
Miserable.
Sad.
Afraid.
Frustrated.
Overwhelmed.
Defeated.
Disappointed.
Undesirable.
Unwell.
Unhappy.
Unaccomplished…

I'm sure there are some other "un" words I'm missing here, but you get the point.

As you read these words, I want you to remember the only time we truly fail is when we stop trying altogether. The fact that you chose this book means that you are STILL trying. You're still here, even after all of those previously heartbreaking attempts that brought you close to your goal -- or maybe even helped you achieve it -- only to lose your footing and slide all the way back to where you started...or maybe even further back than that...

Do you realize how much strength and courage it takes to open up this book and decide to start making positive changes in your life?! It's not easy to keep picking yourself back up over and over again...and yet, here you are-- here WE are--working to change our lives together. And it is this strength, courage, and dedication to not give up on ourselves that will keep driving us toward our goals.

I cannot tell you how freaking excited I am to have you here, reading these pages, RIGHT AT THIS VERY MOMENT! Let me tell you...I was extremely scared to write this book, and I wasn't sure I was *actually* going to follow through with it...but here we are, ready to get this party started. First things first, though... I'm sure you're wondering who is on the other side of these pages, right?! Well, here's a little bit about me...

ALLOW ME TO INTRODUCE MYSELF...

I always have such a hard time writing these "about me" sections...but you're here, and I feel like it would be weird if I tried to help you change your life without telling you a little bit more about myself! My name is Melyssa, and I am a Positive Lifestyle Coach on a mission to make the journey to healthy living accessible, entertaining, and enjoyable! What does a Positive Lifestyle Coach do? My mission is to help you figure out your strengths, build your motivation and confidence through powerful questions and reflections, and help you set goals and develop action plans for your success! As I mentioned briefly above, my job as a coach is not to tell you what to do but to help you figure out what YOU want to do and HOW you want to do it!

In my professional life, I am a board-certified lifestyle medicine professional and certified health and well-being coach. I'm also a group fitness instructor and hold a master's in clinical psychology from the University of Central Florida (*Go Knights, Charge On!*). In addition, I've held numerous roles in my post-graduate career, including a registered mental health counseling intern; a wellness manager at an inpatient substance use treatment center; a clinician well-being coach at a large healthcare organization; and a health educator at an even LARGER (*and competing*) healthcare organization.

So that's the fancy and formal introduction, but, on a more personal note, I am a...
-dedicated dog mom to my senior golden lab, Buddy;
-multi-passionate entrepreneur;
-lover of vanilla-hazelnut iced lattes;
-sucker for a resort-style pool;
-recovering perfectionist;
-passionate group fitness instructor;
-wannabe back-up dancer for Beyonce and Lizzo;
-Jill-of-all-trades, master of none;

-classy and badass-y lady with a sailor's mouth (*that's right, folks, you can be BOTH!*);
-world-champion bully to myself;
-person who constantly finds herself on the "is it undiagnosed ADD or a trauma response?" side of the social media algorithms (*personally, I'm convinced it's both*);
-hot mess of healing from previous emotional abuse;
-advocate for breaking generational traumas;
-survivor of my own trauma;
-chronic worrier;
-chronic illness warrior;
-work in progress and a masterpiece simultaneously (*just like we all are!*);
-person who starts **MANY** things...and finishes only a few
-self-sabotaging, imposter syndrome battling, personal development junkie;
-consistently inconsistent change maker;
-Ph.D. program dropout;
-friend who forgets to send birthday cards and gifts...I know, it's the worst–I really do need to work on this...;
-someone who lived her childhood dream job as a marine mammal trainer.

Now, I like to say that I went from training animals to training humans! (*And if you ask my friends...they will tell you that joke gets old after a while...*) My animal training career helped me develop effective public speaking skills (*there's nothing like having to improvise in front of thousands of people while working with animals...!*), extensive knowledge of behavior modification (*just FYI, I no longer use belly rubs or fish as reinforcement for my clients*), and a passion for inspiring people to change their lives to support wildlife conservation. And now, my new passion is inspiring positive lifestyle transformations for individuals so they can become their happiest, healthiest selves.

However, as I write this introduction, I feel like I'm in the worst health of my life. I am the heaviest I've ever weighed and also the weakest I've been in a very long time with my cardiovascular endurance and muscular strength. I am on the path to recovery after battling burnout from the COVID-19 pandemic while working in the healthcare industry. If living through that insane time warp also hit you and your well-being harder than ever, please remember, **you're not alone.** And if you find yourself in a setback that wasn't due to the pandemic, that's totally normal too! Let's face it, changing our habits can be HARD!

So...what makes me qualified to take you on this journey? Honestly, I STILL wonder about that sometimes! I mean, sure, I have the technical training through my previous jobs as a personal trainer, mental health counselor, clinician well-being coach, and health educator, but I guess the fact that I am living this journey right alongside you is the real reason why you can trust me! I am at a place in my life right now where I KNOW what I need to be doing for my health and wellness, but I am having a tough time APPLYING that knowledge in my own life...which (obviously) isn't the most helpful approach and isn't going to get the results I desire.

It is often said that we teach what we need to learn most, and at this point in my life, I find that 100% true. I wrote this book because I was having a hard time finding something that I could relate to that:
- included powerful activities to help me gain insight into my thought and behavior patterns

- could touch on sensitive topics while bringing a lighthearted, compassionate energy through shared experiences
- was based on the latest scientific research
- and, lastly, was conversational and didn't make me feel like I was reading a textbook

In this book, I am not only coaching myself through the process of regaining my own health and happiness...but I'm also sharing everything I wish I had known when I was first attempting to be "healthy." So many times, I felt that "health" looked a certain way based on what we see around us in society. But I've come to realize that if we put the energy we use fighting to change our minds and bodies into learning how to work WITH our minds and bodies instead, we could create a life in which we THRIVE! I hope to encourage you to stop being so hard on yourself too.

I also aim to share the basics of healthy living from evidence-based practices like lifestyle medicine, positive psychology, and mindfulness. I will provide you with activities and exercises to put that knowledge into practice. However, I do want to educate you on the latest research because adopting more health-promoting habits can increase our lifespans and reduce our risk of and even prevent certain chronic diseases!

Disclaimer: Let's be perfectly clear, though: I am not a doctor or a licensed mental health provider--and I am definitely not YOUR healthcare provider--so please remember that this book is meant to present only educational information and not medical advice or any kind of clinical diagnosis. Always speak with your primary care provider or a specialist if you have any concerns about your health and well-being.

WHAT TO EXPECT...

If you are anything like me, your mind might be chattering away with thoughts of self-doubt and anticipatory defeat. You might be thinking, *"I've already tried so many things; how is this going to be any different? ...I just can't do it, it's too hard, and I am tired of failing...How am I supposed to find the energy and motivation to make the changes I want in my life? ...I shouldn't even try because I never finish anything...Healthy living DOES suck, and you can't change my mind about that."*

Now, I could keep going with things that my mind is telling me, but, again, we're not here to throw ourselves a pity party or get stuck thinking about everything we've sucked at in the past. So, even though our minds LOOOOOVE to bring those cringe-worthy memories and thoughts up for us over and over again, it's time to move on.

Here's what I am asking you to do as we start this journey together. First, I invite you to give yourself permission to drop the self-imposed struggle of trying to fight your thoughts and feelings. And I'd like you to have an open mind to trying out new ways to create positive and supportive experiences for yourself and to be OK with your "failures" and "mistakes" along the way! Instead of taking the rigid, aggressive, *"I MUST FOLLOW (XYZ) PLAN 100%"* approach," I'd like you to try the curious, appreciative, *"I'm a researcher, and I am my own experiment"* approach.

In fact, as you're moving through this book, it should become evident that phrases like, "All you need to do is what I did...just try this quick fix..." are a BIIIIG red flag! Now, I'm not telling you NOT to listen to other people, but I am telling you to take what they say with a healthy amount of skepticism. That includes what I say too! I don't want you to have blind faith in me just because I am writing the book on how to make healthy living NOT suck. This book is a walkthrough experience to help YOU find what works best for YOU to create lasting changes.

That means you will need to try out some of the skills I'll be sharing and have patience through the process. Remember, we are in this for the long haul, not the overnight success, which doesn't exist anyway... Lastly, give yourself permission to try new things and fail at them...because that will give us invaluable information as you go along your journey.

In this journey together, we are going to face the hard truths, work to figure out how we can best help ourselves accomplish our goals, and, ultimately, begin building a foundation of behaviors that support health in creating a life where you thrive! My wish for you (and myself!) is to establish these sustainable habits, so they become part of your lifestyle and don't take as much brain power or willpower... This will allow you to use your energy to do what you love with the people you care about most!

I am most excited to bring you this book because I LITERALLY CANNOT WAIT to hear your success stories as we go through this journey together! So, as I sit at my desk, sipping my coffee and watching my sweet doggo asleep at my feet, I imagine the future letters I will get from you, my readers. I can't wait to hear how you've reclaimed your health and transformed your lifestyle with positive habits...I can't help but get giddy thinking about it!

You have to promise to share your successes with me along the way, okay? *Pinky promise…?* YAAAAS! I'll do the same thing as I continue writing this book to help you remember that you are a human, not a robot.

THIS IS HOW WE DO IT
(*THIS IS HOW WE DO IT!*)

Throughout this book, I'll present different elements to help you gain knowledge, boost your confidence and motivation, and apply the information through activities.

- **EDUCATE**: These sections will introduce relevant information on how changing your habits around a particular topic will help you feel happier and healthier.
- **EMPOWER**: These sections will guide you through activities to increase your motivation and build your confidence to change.
- **ENGAGE**: These sections will provide relevant practices for you to work through the skills being taught. They will also include behavior trackers for you to use for your own behavior change goals.

Okay, my Change Makers – are we ready to get started?! I hope you answered with an enthusiastic **LET'S DO THIS!** and are excited to build some positive momentum! But, before we get started working on what we want to change, the first thing we need to do is find our…

"YOU ARE HERE" Sticker!

Chapter 1:
"You are HERE!"

"The journey of a thousand miles
begins with a single step."
—*Lao Tzu*

Now that you've had the chance to learn about me, I'd love to get to know the "you" on the other side of the pages! But, more importantly, I want to invite you to take some time getting to know YOU – the you that is right here, right now. The YOU that is the changemaker holding this book and reading these pages. Getting to know ourselves again has to be the first part of our journey together. Through this process, we can take a good, long look in the mirror and get honest about accepting where we are starting and figuring out where we want to go.

Admittedly, I'm having a hard time sharing my starting point with you. It's a challenge for me because I feel like I have fallen sooo far from where I worked SOOOOO incredibly hard to get to before. In graduate school, I worked out regularly and taught group fitness classes (*my endurance and strength were better than EVER!*). I was eating well, even on a student budget, had a solid morning routine with meditation and journaling, and felt confident with how I looked and satisfied with my career.

Fast forward to the start of the pandemic. While my eating habits spiraled out of control, I started drinking more alcohol than ever. I still occasionally taught virtual fitness classes, but I blew off my own workouts, and, over time, less and less of my clothes fit properly. My routines were thrown out of whack, and I began feeling overwhelmed and dissatisfied. I also started questioning what I was working toward as I kept finding myself in "bait-and-switch" jobs, which led to a lack of fulfillment in my work. Thankfully, I have slowly but surely been working my way out of that downward spiral!

So where am I starting now, then? Luckily, I've found a job I LOVE with an incredible team doing meaningful work every day. I'm slowly but surely bringing back my morning routine habits, and since I work remotely, I'm also creating a new structure for my workday that best supports me. In addition, my nutrition has improved, and I'm getting back to teaching fitness classes again, which is helping me battle my insecurities and body image issues. I am proud of my progress so far, but I also know I have a long way to go before reaching some of the BIG goals I've set for myself!

If anyone knows how much it can suck to sit here and reflect on where you're starting, it's YA GIRL right here. Like I shared in the introduction, I have been a total avoidance queen when it comes to this. I know I am not happy with where I am...but the more I turn a blind eye to acknowledging and accepting that this is where I'm at, the less likely I am to make changes to help me bust out of this rut. So please know that I'm not asking you to be excited or happy about admitting where we're starting – acceptance does NOT mean approval. But this is the first step in finding the **You Are HERE** sticker for our journey to positive change.

To find your own **You Are HERE** starting point–and to begin designing your Life Map–please take some time now to walk through the following reflection prompts.

EMPOWER

Who I am right now…

Who I want to become…

What I need to do to become my desired future self…

Wellness Wheel:
This reflection activity allows you to take a compassionate look in the metaphorical "mirror" and explore your satisfaction (on a scale of 0-10) with different areas of your life. I've included a few suggestions of some areas of well-being to consider, but feel free to use whichever categories fit best for YOU! I would encourage you to use this tool to measure how your life satisfaction begins to change as you make positive lifestyle changes.

- Traditional Eight Dimensions of Wellness include: *Physical, Intellectual, Emotional, Social, Spiritual, Occupational, Financial, and Environmental.*
- Other Suggested Life Areas could include: *Family, Leisure, Mental, Personal Growth, Intimacy, or Parenting.*

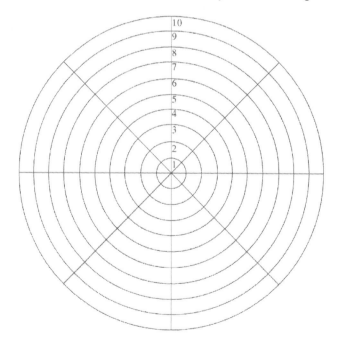

What do you feel is already going well for you from your wellness wheel activity?

What are the top three life areas from your wellness wheel that you would like to improve?

I would rate my current level of overall health and well-being as…

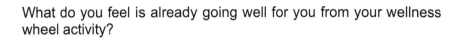

      0 - 1 - 2 - 3 - 4 - 5 - 6 - 7 - 8 - 9 - 10
(*very poor*)   (*excellent*)

- Why did you choose the number above and not a lower number?

What are you hoping to gain from reading this book and working through the activities?

EDUCATE

"Your beliefs become your thoughts,
Your thoughts become your words,
Your words become your actions,
Your actions become your habits,
Your habits become your values,
Your values become your destiny."

– Mahatma Gandhi

Values, Goals, and Habits…OH MY!

Now that we've taken some time to reflect on where we are starting and the direction we would like our journey to take, we need to better understand how lifestyle behaviors connect to our values, goals, and habits. In fact, these components help create our "Life Map." It might seem like common sense as you read through this section, but this reflection is a crucial part of creating awareness of your patterns, connecting to your reasons for change, and continuing to learn from any slip-ups that might happen along the way.

Since this is *your* journey, *you* need to decide where you want to go! Think about it this way: if you were going somewhere you've never been before, wouldn't you want a map to know whether you're going in the right direction? It's certainly helpful to have directions and landmarks you can refer to along the way to let you know you are on the right track! You can think of your values as the compass, your goals as the GPS, and your habits as the actions you take when following or disregarding the GPS directions.

Let's now look at each of the elements to see how they play into your lifestyle change journey...

VALUES

Values are like the compass on your Life Map. Your values give you direction toward your "North," but you never actually reach a destination called "North." They provide you with constant guidance and help you decide how you want to live your life. Everyone's values will look different, and, chances are, your values might have changed during the different phases of your life, too. For example, while I was in elementary through high school, one of my values was Intelligence. I always wanted to strive for the highest grades possible! As I moved into college, Intelligence became less important to me and was eventually replaced by Love of Learning. While my grades were still important to me, I became more focused on the knowledge I was gaining and how I could apply it in my future career.

Your values might have shifted as well over time. Maybe at one point in your life, you were focused on excelling in your career, so the values of Hard Work, Dedication, and Being Driven were most important. But then, as you started a family, the values of Presence, Love, and Care shifted into a higher priority. The good news is no one value is better than another--your preferences are more about how *you* want your life to look and feel.

Once you identify your values, you can use them as a compass to give you direction in life and to help you make more helpful choices. But if you don't take the time to reflect on and connect with your values, you might just end up wandering around aimlessly through life! Being clear with and connected to your values can help you act aligned with your values even when you don't "feel like it." This alignment is what we call *committed action* – because your *actions* are *committed* to your values regardless of how you feel.

**Spoiler alert: You will quickly learn that you cannot rely solely on your feelings of motivation, inspiration, etc. to make lasting changes. In fact, our feelings can often get in the way of our progress towards change!

GOALS

While our values act as a compass and help us decide on the direction of our journey and which qualities we would like to embody and live by, it is our goals that help us reach various destinations on our Life Map. That is the major difference between a value and a goal: the latter represents a destination we can reach, an actual "finish line." Thinking back to our Life Map, accomplishing a goal is like reaching one of the checkpoints on your journey to change!

Now, maybe you meet your goal fully and arrive at that checkpoint, and you get to say, *"Yes, I did it! I reached my goal!"* Or maybe you get close to reaching your goal--not exactly in the right location on your Life Map, but maybe a few blocks away--and you get to say, *"Wow, I made a lot of progress this time around! I learned a lot while I worked on this goal that can help me with my next goal."* (*And if you have perfectionistic tendencies, you might be pissed you didn't reach your exact destination… later, we will talk about how this type of thinking hinders our change journey.*)

But, then, there might also be times when you are waaaaay off base, and you don't even get close to your checkpoint! Maybe you're not even in the same town…! When that happens, you might be reeeally hard on yourself and beat yourself up or feel disappointed and defeated. Then, all that negative self-talk might start bubbling up, and you might find yourself saying, *"Oh my gosh, I'm SUCH a failure! I can't believe I couldn't do it…This goal was supposed to be so easy, and I still failed… I'm such a loser!"*

That's when you have to pause and say to yourself, *"Oh man…I was really trying this time…and this ain't easy! But that's okay because I'm going to take this experience and try to see what I can learn from it!"* So with any of the goals you don't accomplish, I'd like to encourage you to focus on treating these instances as an opportunity to learn more about yourself! That's the beauty in viewing yourself as your own experiment: you can never TRULY fail, but you CAN learn what won't work to get you the outcome you were hoping for!

TYPES OF GOALS
- **Outcome goal:** A goal focused on a specific *outcome*, just like the name implies! Examples include losing X number

of pounds, fitting into X-size pants, or winning a race. You're focusing on the final product with outcome goals, so they are typically more long-term. However, since outcome goals are the ones we have the **least** amount of control over, we also need to set shorter-term goals along the way that are not outcome-focused.

- **Performance goal:** A goal focused on improving your *performance* with an activity. It can help you notice and measure your progress over time. Examples include improving your running pace or lifting heavier dumbbells while doing strength training exercises.

- **Process goal:** A goal focused on the actual *process* involved in achieving the desired change. Process goals are truly where the magic happens because they allow you the most control over the "finish point." Examples include eating one additional serving of fruit or vegetables during each meal for a week or walking four days per week to improve cardiovascular fitness. WHOA! Did you notice what just happened there?! Framing goals in this way creates smaller ACTION-focused goals that can help you reach your outcome-based long-term goals! So especially when you have a longer term goal, like weight loss, make sure you are focusing on the processes to help you achieve those outcomes.

  - *As a side note—if you are embarking on a weight loss journey, please don't let the scale be your only measure of success! Listen y'all, one pound of fat and one pound of muscle weight the exact same— ONE POUND! So your body composition may be changing and you may be shedding fat and gaining muscle, but the numbers on the scale might not budge! So please make sure you are using other measures of progress that can more accurately reflect changes in your body composition—like waist-to-hip ratios, noticing how your clothes are fitting, etc.*

OK—rant over; let's get back on track!

HABITS

Finally, there are habits. These are the actions you take that align you with your goals! The habits you engage in either help or hinder your progress toward your goals. So, if the habits you created over your lifetime are not positive, it could be extremely difficult to accomplish some of your goals. Here's what I want you to remember, though: Habits are *LEARNED* over time. This is great news because that also means you can *UNLEARN* habits that don't fit your desired lifestyle while you learn new habits that support your health and well-being!

However, I must caution you. While changing your habits can get at the root of making lasting behavior changes, the actual process may prove challenging since habits are the actions you take when you're on "autopilot." Think back to when you learned to tie your shoes or brush your teeth. Those actions required a lot of brain power and focus at the time. Now, though, I'm guessing you could probably do those tasks with your eyes closed, thanks to your muscle memory! This happened because all those movement repetitions eventually became ingrained in your brain. That's pretty cool, right?! That means your brain can now use its energy for other things besides focusing on those behaviors that are part of your routine.

And let's be perfectly clear: I call bullshit on the whole, "*It takes 21 days to create a new habit!*" Realistically, it can take a hell of a lot longer than that because, sometimes, you must undo decades of repetition of a certain habit first. So, I think it should be more like 63 days: 21 days to start breaking the old habit, 21 days to start introducing the new habit, and another 21 days to establish the new habit! The point is there is no "one size fits all" approach to change because we are all different! Not to mention, some habits took years to form–which means trying to break those habits likely won't happen overnight either! Since habits are learned, and we all learn in different ways, it's going to take some investigation to find what works best for you to make positive changes!

The first step in changing habits is becoming aware of the habits you want to LET GO and the habits you want to GROW. The habits you want to LET GO are the ones that pull you further away from your values, while the habits you want to GROW push you closer toward your values. By understanding how your habits work, you will be able to identify where you can intervene in the Habit Loop.

What is the Habit Loop, you ask? GREAT QUESTION! I'd love to tell you.

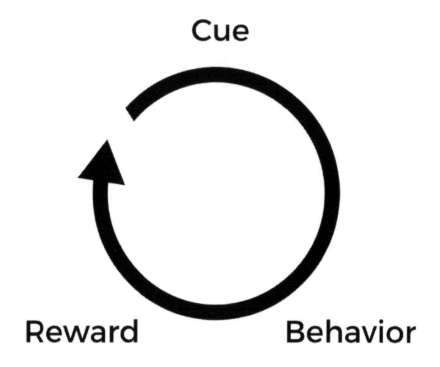

The Habit Loop consists of three components: Cue, Behavior, and Reward. First, a Cue activates the Habit Loop, which then leads to a Behavior or a routine. Then, once you've engaged with the behavior, a Reward follows. The Reward triggers the parts of your brain that say, *"YAY, LET'S DO THAT AGAIN"* after releasing a flood of neurotransmitters like dopamine, further reinforcing the Cue and the Behavior!

It's almost like there is a little dopamine addict living in our brain, seeking out those activities that will give us a "hit" of the good stuff! Of course, I don't say that to minimize the serious issue of addiction. Rather, I'm trying to provide context for understanding the vicious cycle created through these reward pathways in your brain. As soon as you're exposed to a Cue, the Habit Loop gets activated, and you immediately crave the reward that comes from engaging in that particular Behavior.

Here is the good news—we have the ability to "retrain our brain" when it comes to habits! The science-y term for this awesome phenomenon is "neuroplasticity," which basically means we can create new neural pathways in our brains over time! This is helpful to know because it should give you hope and help you feel empowered that YOU CAN CHANGE.

There's a common phrase among the science world that goes like this: *Neurons that fire together, wire together.* What that boils down to is the more you practice something, the stronger those neural pathways in the brain grow! And the less we engage in the habits we want to let go of, those pathways will begin to wear down over time and the automaticity of the unhelpful behavior fades. That means the more you engage in habits you want to grow in your life, those pathways will get "etched" into your brain until it becomes part of your routine!

Let's walk through a personal example of mine to better understand how the Habit Loop works. I tend to be a mindless snacker, especially when I'm on the couch in front of the television. As a family, my parents and I ALWAYS ate dinner in front of the TV, creating a strong association between watching TV and eating. Consequently, watching TV on the couch eventually became a Cue for me, leading to the Behavior of eating – even when I wasn't hungry! My Reward was the feeling I had when I munched on something delicious while enjoying my favorite show or watching a movie.

Eventually, this became a pattern of behavior that I wasn't even paying much attention to. I'd keep munching until I found myself at the bottom of the bag of potato chips, wondering where they all went! That's because once a behavior is established in the Habit Loop, there's not much brain power dedicated to it anymore. You end up in autopilot mode, just going through the motions! This autopilot mode is one of the biggest challenges to changing habits. We are often unaware we're engaging in the undesired behavior until afterward, when we're like,"*SHIT, how did I let this happen again?!*" The realization is then typically followed by a flurry of unhelpful thoughts or upsetting emotions like guilt, shame, or embarrassment.

It's going to take some intentional attention—and some planning in advance—to start chipping away at that established Habit Loop and building new patterns. But I hope having a better understanding of the Habit Loop helps you feel more empowered in recognizing that we CAN change our habits. We will take a closer look at some of the strategies that can help us let go of old habits and grow new ones in the next section.

Now that you've got a better understanding of how values, goals, and habits are connected to lifestyle changes, I'd like to walk you through activities to help you explore your own values, set effective goals, and hack your habits!

EMPOWER

VALUES EXPLORATION: CREATING YOUR COMPASS

If you are reading this book, chances are, your health and well-being are important to you! Being able to really dive into these life areas to figure out what your ideal scenario looks like will give you a sense of direction for your actions and choices. Values are not fixed–and they vary from person to person–so revisiting your values frequently will help you continue living a fulfilled life!

What's important to you? What do you value in your life? What brings value to your life? How (What?) do you want to "be" in the world? What qualities do you want to reflect?

BEING A GOAL-GETTER

Setting effective goals is extremely important when it comes to successful and lasting lifestyle changes. I'd like you to take a moment to think about a goal you've had in the past–specifically, a goal you didn't accomplish. First, think about...

- What happened to keep you from reaching the goal?
- What threw you off track? What did it look like?
- Were there some thoughts that contributed to not following through with the goal?

Next, I invite you to think about...

- What went well during that time?
- Did you fail at every attempt at that goal?
- Were you able to accomplish any smaller steps of the process that moved you toward your big goal?

As you worked through the prompts above, what did you learn? What information did you gain from this reflection activity that you can use to support you when setting new goals?

Usually, you can have SOME success while working towards a goal, even if just for that initial time when you're PUMPED and motivated to accomplish it. But then, your motivation might start fading. You might start making excuses and promising yourself you'll just try again next year, when it's time to make New Year's resolutions. I think we've AAALLLLLLL been there before!

When you don't accomplish a goal, I think it's important to reflect on what didn't work out and, also, what went WELL during the process! It's the perfect time to ask yourself: Was that goal too ambitious right off the bat? Did it feel overwhelming? Or, perhaps, you had already convinced yourself you couldn't reach it, and then it became almost like a self-fulfilling prophecy of, "*I'm never going to be able to reach this goal, so why even try?!*" Or, maybe, you've missed a day or two, and don't feel like it makes sense to keep going...even though it totally does!

When those instances happen, I think you have an opportunity to strengthen your self-awareness by reflecting on what went wrong in a patient, curious, and compassionate way. That reflection becomes your superpower. At some point, you begin to understand yourself SOOO much that you can now focus on learning to overcome similar challenges or obstacles the next time you encounter them. Basically, you learn how to become your own coach through those challenges instead of getting stuck or falling back into old routines.

Tips for Setting Effective Goals:
- **Connect them to your values.** Remind yourself of the importance of the goal and your reasons for wanting to make the change. Come back to the WHY behind your desired changes to reconnect with the meaning behind your actions.
- **Focus on framing your goals positively (adding something in) versus negatively (taking something away).** The more you try to deprive or restrict yourself of something, the more you crave it because it feels forbidden! Instead, set your sights on the positive changes you want to add to your life.
- **Don't set a "dead person's" goal.** This means if a dead person can do it better than you, don't use that goal! This usually refers to the "nevers" and "won'ts"–like "*never*

drinking soda again" or "I *won't* eat sugar anymore." While there aren't zombies out there (*at least that I know of!*) downing some sodas or popping some chocolates, you get the idea–don't be too drastic or strict with your goals!

- **Focus on only one to three small goals at a time to prevent overwhelm.** Instead of trying to half-ass a bunch of different goals, put your ENTIRE ASSES into a small set of goals!
- **Make them action-oriented and behavior-driven.** You may be tempted to set goals like "feel happier" or "feel less stressed," but you need to focus on actual actions and behaviors that can help you experience those desired emotional states.
- **Keep your goals flexible.** Allow your goals to be a "living document" so that you can make adjustments as needed. The more rigid you are with your goals, the more likely you are to give up instead of modifying them to support your success!
- **Set time frames of weeks, months, and years.** You want to have a mix of long-term and short-term goals to create a sense of urgency AND to have plenty of checkpoints on your Life Map!

Setting SMART Goals

Chances are you may have seen the SMART goals framework somewhere before–working with a personal trainer, at a corporate training, in a leadership development class, etc. The reason this method of goal setting is so popular is that it has been scientifically supported for setting effective goals regardless of the setting. This model works well because you have to be clear about what you are working on and how you will measure it. It also connects your goal to a dedicated timeline. Let's see how this all comes together in the SMART acronym below...

S–What specific behavior/action are you focusing on?
Setting vague goals like, "*I want to improve my health and well-being*," without any specifics on what that improvement looks like, is like deciding you want to make a recipe and not having a list of ingredients or directions for how to make it! When you set your goals, you must get specific to have clarity and direction for a successful behavior change. So be sure to choose a specific action or behavior for the main focus of your goal.

M–Measurable: How will you measure it?
Deciding how you will measure your behavior change gives you an opportunity to check in and say, "*Did I meet this goal?*" You could measure your goal based on duration of time, frequency of sessions, distance, etc.

A–Achievable: How will you set yourself up for success?
Making sure that you have the resources you need to achieve this goal ahead of time can increase your chances of success. You could create a system for yourself, get additional support or resources, or take steps to build in reminders for your goal.

R–Realistic: How confident are you that you can achieve this goal?
This is where I like to do a confidence test on a scale of zero (not at all confident, never gonna happen!) to ten (absolutely! 100%! Not a doubt in my mind!). You want to be somewhere between seven and nine on the confidence scale. That score means you believe you can achieve the goal, but it's juuuust challenging enough for you without feeling overwhelming! If your confidence is

at a ten, the goal is too easy for you – you could add a bit of a challenge in there! And if it's at a six or below, you might need to reassess the goal or see what could give you a confidence boost– and remember, it's okay to change your goals! Think of your goals as "living documents" that you can revisit, readjust, and reassess as needed.

T–Time-Bound: When will you do this goal, and for how long?
Creating a timeline for sticking to the goal is very important. You could set a starting date, decide to do the goal on certain days of the week, or resolve to do it for a certain number of months before building onto it. You want to have some sense of time connected to your goals to create urgency and help you stay accountable to follow through!

EXAMPLE: I will walk (S) around the neighborhood for 45 minutes (M) with my neighbor (A), twice a week at 7am on Mondays and Thursdays for the next 4 weeks (T). My confidence level is an eight (R).

Write Yourself a "Lifestyle Prescription."
This is another method of goal setting that you might find helpful because you get to "prescribe" a behavior to yourself!
- **F - Frequency:** How often will you do this behavior?
- **I - Intensity:** How long will you do this behavior?
- **T - Time:** When will you do this behavior?
- **T - Type**: What is the behavior?
- **EXAMPLE:**
  - F: 3 days per week, I: 5 minutes, T: before getting ready for bed, T: gratitude journal

Changing Your Habits

I invite you to think about some of your current habits - everything from brushing your teeth to having your morning cup of coffee. Do not classify these as "good/bad" habits; just take a quick inventory of ALL the habits you can identify.

Current Habits

Was there anything on this list that surprised you? Isn't it crazy how many things we DO throughout the day without even realizing it at times!? Now, take a moment to write out which habits from the list you want to LET GO and which ones you want to GROW. Your desired habits may or may not be listed above, so feel free to add whichever ones you'd like to have in your life.

LET GO	GROW

Okay, now that you know WHAT habit changes you want to make, let's talk about HOW to actually do that...

Habits you want to GROW: When creating new habits, you need to remember that patience and attention are crucial! You've taken the steps to identify which positive habits you want to build into your life, and now you're going to learn the skills to get this habit to stick!

- **Get Your Reps In!** Since habits are learned through repetition, you need to work your mental muscles through reps at your "mental fitness" gym! You have to practice the new behavior (many times? frequently?) to strengthen those mental muscles that will help it become a habit! Remember, you're not looking for perfection here – every repetition you get in is progress!

- **Get a Cue!** Here's one way to hack your Habit Loop: create a cue for your new habit! Whether it's a sticky note on your laptop telling you to drink water or a reminder on your phone set for your daily meditation, choose something simple as a cue for the new behavior! Eventually, as your habit becomes more ingrained into your routine, your environment will serve as your cue, and you may not need those additional reminders anymore! But you can always reintroduce cues as needed because it can be easy to slip back into those old patterns over time!

- **Treat Yo'self!** It feels GOOD to follow through with something you intend to do, doesn't it?! Each and every time you complete your new habit, you should celebrate! This is going to help reinforce your new behavior AND your cue for the behavior. Rewards promote the formation of new habits. So even small celebrations--like giving yourself a high five, a pat on the back, or some words of encouragement–even if they feel silly at first, will set off the reward circuitry in your brain and release all those neurotransmitters that tell us, "*OOOO! We liked that! Let's* *do it again!*" Yet another way we can hack our Habit Loop and build that positive momentum toward change!

Habits you want to LET GO: It can be challenging to break old habits, but only because we spend so much of our time in autopilot mode! And if we don't even realize we're engaging in these habits, it's going to be hella hard to let them go. Here are some ways we can promote breaking those old habits to make room for our fresh, new ones:

- **Change it Up!** Could you remove the cue, change something in your environment to avoid the cue, or make a healthier swap?? Being able to restructure your surroundings can help support positive change too! This one works wonders for my mindless munching in front of the TV habit:
  - If I don't have a bag of chips to snack on, then POOF, they can't magically disappear when I'm watching TV!
  - I can also avoid bringing the bag of chips over to the couch and use a smaller bowl to portion out some chips. That way, I reach the bottom of a bowl instead of the bottom of an entire bag!
  - I could also decide to nosh on some carrots and hummus as my munchy-crunchy TV snack. I can still enjoy myself, but the carrots are a much healthier option than chips!
- **STOP!** This trick helps you interrupt the Habit Loop by creating some space for yourself after encountering a cue by literally saying STOP. You can also use any other variation of a word/phrase that will make you pause: WAIT! TIME-OUT! WHOA THERE! This action will help you disrupt the Habit Loop activation BEFORE engaging in the

behavior that follows the cue. Will you avoid the behavior every time you practice this? Most likely not, but that's okay! Because even recognizing the cue in the first place is a great way to work towards change as it helps you identify your space to make a choice.

- **Make a choice!** You have the ability to create a magical space between the Cue and the Behavior on the Habit Loop to stop yourself from falling into mindlessness! Stopping yourself after you've encountered a Cue allows you to recognize the choices and actions that either *pull you further away* from or *push you closer toward* your values. You want to monitor your choices so you can celebrate **each and every time** you make a choice that supports your goals or learn from the times you make a choice that moves you further away from your goals.

Take some time now to reflect on a habit of yours:

Cue(s):

Behavior:

Reward(s):

What are some barriers (obstacles/challenges) you have encountered in your life before?

What has worked well for you in the past in overcoming these barriers?

What are some barriers to change that you anticipate running into again?

How can you avoid/work around/move past those barriers this time?

Take some time to write out your Life Map. Imagine accomplishing all the changes you want to make and living aligned with your values to become your desired future self. What would you be doing? How would you be feeling? What does your day-to-day look like? What will you have accomplished?

As you build positive habits, there will be times when you fall back into old patterns or miss an opportunity to practice your new habit – and that's okay! Remember, this is all just an experimental process to find what works best for YOU. And as you try new things, you need to give them a fighting chance too! Don't just try a habit once and be like, "*Eh, this isn't going to work for me....*" Instead, keep that open-minded curiosity I talked about earlier and try new things, gather information and insight, and build your lifestyle change toolbox!

PHEW! How are you feeling about everything so far? If you're still noticing that nagging voice reminding you of all your failed attempts or saying you won't be able to do this, refocus on the words on this page and let your mind chatter away in the background! You want to remember, as the great Tony Robbins says, "where focus goes, energy flows." So if you're focusing on the thoughts that hold you back, you will stay stuck. But if you notice that you've gotten sucked in by negativity, you can refocus back to your desired Life Map!

I know, I know, this is ALL a lot easier said than done...but we're going to take the next step in recognizing that...

Chapter 2:

MINDSET MATTERS

If one advances confidently in the direction of his dreams, and endeavors to live the life which he has imagined, he will meet with a success unexpected in common hours.

–Henry David Thoreau

Our minds can either work for us or against us, especially if we are not paying careful attention to the mental chatter happening in our brains. Even more so when we are doing our best to make changes and get caught up in our self-critical thoughts. The more aware we become of our thought patterns, the more aware we become of how our thoughts affect our behaviors.

Listen Change Makers, if anyone knows how much your mind can either work FOR you or AGAINST you, it is definitely yours truly! OK...here we go with the vulnerability...*audible GULP.*

I've struggled with anxiety, bouts of depression, post-traumatic stress disorder, complicated grief, disordered eating, and body dysmorphia. And I'm sure I'm missing something from that list too. It has been an UGLY and SUPER UNCOMFORTABLE healing process, but the journey has ABSOLUTELY been worth it. And you may be thinking, *"YIKES...didn't Melyssa say she has experience as a mental health counselor...?"* Yup, you remembered correctly! And yes, I want to normalize seeing a therapist that goes to therapy. In fact, it may even be one of the healthiest things a therapist can do for their own well-being! So, even though I read the textbooks, had the training, and worked with clients with similar challenges in life, it is wonderful to spend time in sessions as the client myself. Therapy allows me to learn how to live a fulfilled life with those conditions in the passenger seat of my life instead of in the driver's seat.

All of that is to say that if you feel like you've struggled your entire life, please know I get it. But this book is meant to help us stop struggling, embrace our experiences, and learn how to work WITH our bodies and minds to create lasting lifestyle changes. So does that mean everything is on the up and up from here on out?

Well, as much as I wish that were the case, I'd be lying to you if I said that every day would be great (even good) once you've started your transformation journey.

Let's talk about how the way we think about ourselves affects our chances of success, shall we? Listen, you probably have that inner drill sergeant voice screaming at you, *"PUT DOWN THAT THIRD SLICE OF PIZZA, FATASS! WHY WOULD YOU EVEN TRY TO LOSE WEIGHT AGAIN IF YOU ALWAYS JUST GAIN IT BACK ANYWAYS?! YOU'RE FAT. YOU'RE ALWAYS GOING TO BE FAT. AND UNLESS YOU LOSE WEIGHT, NOBODY IS GOING TO WANT TO BE WITH YOU!"* Ouch! Did reading that hurt you as much as writing it hurt me? These are just some of the many phrases my inner "mean girl" LOVES to throw at me when I am feeling my worst but trying my best. Your inner critic phrases may sound completely different based on the stories you've told yourself, but I'm sure they sting just as much as my examples above.

Okay, okay...I can already hear some of you thinking, *"But Melyssa, that's how I keep myself motivated! I won't stay accountable if I don't have those thoughts!"* Yeah, I know that you might believe that's the only way to keep yourself motivated to change, but let me ask you this: how well has that worked for you in the past?? If the negative self-talk has somehow worked for you, I'm going to take a wild guess and say it was probably temporary. Most likely, you were miserable through the process of trying to change, before you fell back into old patterns of behavior and thought to yourself, *"You loser... I knew you couldn't do it...."*

I know how much it sucks and hurts to find yourself in that dark place, but I also know that there is another way. A way that will not only help you change but also transform your relationship with yourself. We will get to that part in the next chapter, but first, we need to tackle those unhelpful thoughts!

EDUCATE

Believe it or not, many of us have a habit of thinking a certain way! Typically, our thought patterns are influenced by various life events. What's important to remember, though, is that just like we can learn new habits, we can also learn new thought patterns by "retraining our brains," thanks to neuroplasticity!

GROWTH VS. FIXED MINDSET

Before we get any deeper, we need to discuss the concept of mindset. Mindset–defined by Dr. Carol Dweck, Stanford University psychologist–is your unique perspective that determines how you live your life, see the world, and make decisions. Dr. Dweck's work discusses the idea of a fixed mindset versus a growth mindset. It also explores how our thoughts about ourselves affect the world around us and how they influence our performance.

So if we want to make significant changes in our lives, we gotta ditch the fixed mindset thinking patterns! I hate to break it to you, but, chances are, you WILL fail at some point. You might also want to quit, throw your hands in the air and scream a great big, *"WHAT THE FUCK!"* after life blindsides you with a bitch slap that stings like no other! But should we throw away any and all progress we might have made along the way whenever we slip up? How would that be helpful?! *Spoiler alert: it would NOT!*

To better understand what fixed and growth mindset thoughts look like, let's take a look at some examples:

FIXED	GROWTH
I can't do that…	I can practice getting better at that!
They're just smarter than I am…	I know I can improve if I find the support I need to learn this!
I'm so jealous they can do that; I'll never be able to…	It is inspiring to see someone accomplish that! It motivates me to work even harder!
If I fail, I should just quit trying…	Failing means I'm trying something new, and I can learn something from each of my attempts!

It's time for us to choose a new way of tackling our lifestyle change journey. We need to learn to give ourselves permission to fuck up along the way! C'mon, say it with me (*if you're not currently around small children*):

I'm going to fuck up sometimes, and that's OK!
I give myself permission to fuck up and learn from my fuck ups moving forward!

DAAAYUUUM! How GOOD did that feel?!

If we don't learn to cultivate a growth mindset that supports success, we are going to make this lifestyle change journey a *HELLUVA* lot harder on ourselves! And while our minds mean well, our thoughts and the patterns of thinking we develop over time might hold us back from progressing toward the life we desire. While we can't completely control our thoughts, we CAN change how we think about our thoughts.

The fancy name for "thinking about our thoughts" is metacognition, which some believe is what sets us apart from other mammals. Although, after being outsmarted by a few clever animals during my time as a trainer, I'm not so sure that we are the ONLY mammals with this ability...Regardless, we can learn how to relate to our thoughts differently based on how we think about them.

The reason we need to have a discussion about the power of our thoughts is that they can have a significant impact on our behavior. So allow me to introduce you to the Cognitive Triangle!

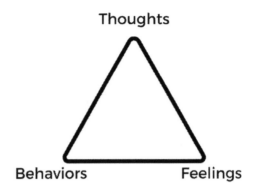

Thoughts

Behaviors   Feelings

This diagram demonstrates the interaction between our thoughts, feelings, and behaviors. From it, we can see that what we think affects how we feel and behave, how we feel affects how we think and behave, and how we behave affects how we feel and think.

COGNITIVE DISTORTIONS

We need to be cautious, though. Because we tend to have common errors in our thought patterns, our feelings and behaviors can be influenced in a way that can keep us from reaching our goals. This, in turn, can make us feel stuck or defeated. These thought errors are referred to as cognitive distortions. They can cause us all sorts of issues if they get in the way of our thinking about the world! As you read through them, you may feel personally attacked by one or more of the categories–I know I always do! Keep in mind, though, that this information is meant to help you overcome self-imposed obstacles and strike down self-sabotaging behavior.

All-or-Nothing Mindset: You guessed it–This mindset refers to the "no gray areas" kind of thinking! When we have the all-or-nothing mindset, we tend to allow our first little mistake to derail us completely. This can also be referred to as "either/or" thinking since we tend to believe things come in absolutes, like you're *either* poor and kind *OR* a rich jackass. But you could also be a rich, kind person or a broke jackass too! So when it comes to our behavior change journey, we need to allow ourselves permission to drop the "either/or" thinking and remember that we have room for the "and" in our lives! You can eat the donut AND still lose weight, binge a show on Netflix AND still get a workout in, have your cake AND eat it too! So when we think we are throwing away all of our progress just because we missed one workout during our 30-day program, we need to remember the "and." After all, it's much easier to allow yourself the rest day and to pick back up where you've left off than to keep restarting a program repeatedly because you've missed a day.

"Should" Statements: My favorite phrase from psychologist Clayton Barbeau is *Stop "shoulding" yourself!* I hope you laughed at the quote because, to me, it means that *"shoulding"* yourself is just as unhelpful as shitting yourself! (*Get it?!*) Constantly thinking, *"I should do this... I shouldn't eat that...Shouldn't I be more motivated?",* usually doesn't help us to take value-committed action. In fact, it only makes us feel worse about ourselves! So, instead of thinking about what you *should* do, think about what you *could* do. Could you go for a 5-minute walk instead of that 30-minute walk you think you *should* be doing? Could you drink one less soda today instead of thinking you *should* stop drinking soda altogether? When you notice that you are *"shoulding"* yourself, try to shift out of asking what you should do and focus on what you **COULD** do instead!

Discounting the Positives: Our brains have this lovely little feature called a negativity bias, which means we are MUCH more likely to remember the negative things that happen to us than the positive ones. The bias is just one of the ways our brains have evolved over time to help us stay alive, and it is a great protective mechanism until the moment we try to change our lives for the better! Imagine that you have a performance review or a school presentation. Even though you receive ten FABULOUS reviews and comments, there's that *one* person who offers rudely critical feedback. Out of the eleven reviews, which is the one you are likely to have burned into your brain afterward?! If you are like the majority of the population, it would be the negative review that gets lodged into the innermost crevices of your brain. There it waits to pop up at the most inconvenient time to remind you, *"Hey, remember that time when...?"* Instead of allowing that one unhelpful thought to hijack our thinking, we need to practice actively focusing our attention on what works well and building our mental muscles of positivity! While not everything will always go according to plan, pay attention to what IS going well for you! One of my favorite practices from life coach and bestselling author Cara Alwill is creating a daily Celebration List. This list can help you take a moment to be proud of all of the things you DID accomplish and stop you from beating yourself up over the things you haven't done yet.

Overgeneralization: When you overgeneralize, you take an isolated incident and apply it to any and all aspects of your life. This thinking error usually contains the absolutes: never, won't, can't, always, etc. When it comes to your well-being journey, these thoughts might sound like, *"Giving up meat will NEVER work for me... I CAN'T do a push-up... I ALWAYS quit before I finish...."* When you catch yourself having these thoughts, remember quitting on day 20 of a 21-day program doesn't mean you will ALWAYS quit everything you start. And yes, that is a personal example that I'll *NEVER* let myself live that down! (*See what I did there; using that word "never"?*)

Magnification: This distortion causes us to blow things WAY out of proportion! Basically, you take an insignificant issue and magnify it into the cliche doomsday scenario of *"the sky is falling!"* When it comes to the behavior change journey, an example of magnification would be assuming that a minor ankle sprain and the following recovery period could undo all of your hard work. While it's true that you might experience a slight setback, it doesn't mean that you're going to lose everything you've worked so hard for! Similarly, giving up on a diet because you've gained a few pounds is an extremely common magnification–but did you know your body weight can fluctuate up to five pounds per day?! So if you gain one pound after having a cupcake at work, chances are it wasn't because of the cupcake–it was probably just your body's normal weight fluctuation. So please *Please* **PLEASE** stop obsessing over the scale!

Minimization: This is when you downplay your accomplishments or minimize yourself in some way. For instance, if someone compliments you on looking more vibrant, you might say, *"Yeah, well, I still have 40 pounds to go until I get to my goal weight."* Who the hell cares?! Obviously, your hard work is paying off if people are taking the time to share their thoughts with you, so don't let yourself downplay your current progress by coming in with a Debbie Downer comment like that (*waaaah waaaaaaah waaaaaaaah–that one is for my SNL fans!*).

Mind Reading: *"Oh my gosh, Elyse didn't wave or smile when I said hello. She must be mad at me for something!"* And cue the downward spiral into the abyss of anxious thinking. Okaaay, yeah, maybe you did something to piss her off.... But what if Elyse simply didn't see or hear you?! Our minds LOVE to try to make sense of all situations, even when we don't have all of the information we need. This is especially true when it comes to our relationships. Our minds end up misinterpreting the slightest miscommunications and turning them into (what feels like) the end of the world!!! So maybe, instead of assuming what someone is thinking, we should just ask and see what they have to say??

Emotional Reasoning: *"I feel like a failure, that must mean I AM a failure."* Just because we feel a certain way in a given moment, doesn't mean we have to allow that feeling to define us forever. This is especially important when it comes to dealing with feelings of motivation. Many times, we may think that just because we don't feel motivated, we don't actually want to accomplish the goal. That is not the case! If you base your entire reasoning on your emotional states, you are going to be ALL over the place when it comes to your behaviors! In the next chapter, we will talk about making some room for our emotions and relating to them in a new way to keep them from being the only driving force behind our behaviors.

Once we begin to recognize our thinking errors, we can choose to relate to those thoughts differently. As I've mentioned before, that recognition can help reduce how much power we give to our thoughts. So, since we can't stop ourselves from having certain thoughts, let's practice some skills to help turn that mental chatter into background noise instead of allowing it to blast so loudly that it keeps us from taking value-committed actions.

EMPOWER

When you take a moment to think back, how many of these thinking errors have you experienced before? Can you think of your own examples in each category?

EDUCATE

YOU ARE NOT YOUR THOUGHTS

We humans have a funny way of letting our thoughts get the best of us sometimes. We can get soooo wrapped up in our thoughts that we make ourselves miserable, sick, and sad! So, since we can't stop ourselves from thinking about certain things, how do we better manage the thoughts our mind throws at us constantly?! Let me introduce you to this method I like to call:

CATCH then CHOOSE or CHANGE

When you *catch* your thinking errors, you can *choose* how you relate to the thought or you can *change* the thought into a more helpful thought! These skills come from the evidence-based approaches of cognitive-behavioral therapy as well as acceptance and commitment training, and can become valuable tools in your well-being toolbox. Since we've already discussed beginning to CATCH our unhelpful thoughts as they happen, let's dive into CHOOSE and CHANGE!

CHOOSE: Getting UNSTUCK from Thoughts

You know when you are putting up a string of decorative holiday lights and find yourself amid a GIANT tangled mess that doesn't seem to have a beginning or an end?! That is a pretty good metaphor for what happens when we get caught up in our thoughts–especially the unhelpful ones. When we get sucked into and all tangled up with our thoughts, we may end up making choices that pull us away from what's important in our lives!

So we want to learn how we can untangle ourselves from the thoughts we have through our CHOOSE skills! Practicing these skills is one of the ways we CHOOSE how to relate differently to the thoughts we have and create space between ourselves and our thoughts, instead of letting ourselves get all tangled up in their mess and engage in behaviors that aren't aligned with our values. The skills that follow are not meant to minimize or dismiss your thoughts at all, but rather to help empower you to recognize that YOU hold power over your thoughts, not the other way around.

Let's take advantage of that awesomely human superpower called metacognition and practice changing the way we think about our thoughts and getting all untangled from that mess we often create for ourselves. Think of these practices like you're trying on a new pair of pants - sometimes they are going to fit comfortably right away, but other times you also may need to wiggle around to stretch them out a bit, or you may not even be able to get them to button up! Again, you have to find what works best for you and give yourself a chance to try on and test out each of these skills.

Notice the thought: Simply creating some space between yourself and your thoughts can be helpful, so let's give this a try now. We've all had some version of the "I'm not good enough" story pop up throughout our lives, and it can feel like a very *heavy* thought. "*I'm not good enough...*" Instead, try thinking that same thought but adding "I'm having the thought that..." in front of it - for example, *I'm having the thought that I'm not good enough.* Notice how that feels a little bit different? It doesn't completely take the sting away, but it helps soften the blow! Let's try and add onto that even more—"*I notice I'm having the thought that I'm not good enough.*" This is a helpful practice for even having us recognize the thoughts as they come up, because we often take our mental chatter as a factual narration of our day, when in reality it is just a biased barrage of thoughts created by our minds.

Slooow it down: Try saying the word *lemon* as slooooowly as you possibly can. Go ahead, give it a try! This technique just brings attention to the fact that words are made up of weird sounds put together! Now try the same thing with an unhelpful thought you have...what happens to the intensity of the thought? If you can take an unhelpful thought and slow it down either in your mind or out loud (maybe not out loud if you're in public somewhere...!), you might be able to take some of the sting away from it!

Speed it up: Similarly to the practice above, try saying the word *lemon* as fast as you can and keep repeating it! Go ahead, as quickly as you can keep saying lemon lemon lemon lemon...! What happened that time? Again, changing the speed of the thought can turn the word or phrase into a big jumble of sounds that don't end up making a lot of sense!

Silly voice: Something that works extremely well for me is thinking the thought in the voice of a character or cartoon–some of my favorite examples are a valley girl voice, Yoda, Patrick Star from Spongebob, and Moira Rose from Schitt's Creek! Notice how the thought of "I'm not good enough" changes when you think the thought in Yoda's voice: "Good enough, I am not!" Everytime I use this example when I'm doing a presentation, the energy in the room shifts and it can even lead to laughter! The context of the thought didn't change at all, but the way we were thinking about it did–which changed how we relate to the original thought.

Sing it: Pairing the thought to a silly song is another way to take some power out of that thought! Let's stick with our example of "I'm not good enough..." Again, that's a pretty heavy thought; definitely doesn't feel good to think that! Now I want you to read this next phrase to the tune of the YMCA chorus: "My mind is telling me–liiiii'm not goooooood ee-nough! My mind is telling mee-eee, liiiii'm not goooooood eee-nouuu-ouuugh!" Oh man, that is one of my FAVORITE techniques to rob a thought of it's hold on me! Other favorable songs for this activity include Happy Birthday, Jingle Bells, Row Row Row Your Boat! I maaaay caution you against using one of your favorite songs for this activity, because you don't want to have that association of your unhelpful thoughts with a song that you enjoy listening to!

Visualize letting go of the thoughts: If you're more of a visual person like me, you may enjoy an activity where you imagine letting go of your thoughts. One of the classic meditations for this is called Leaves on a Stream, where you allow yourself to sit with your thoughts while visualizing a stream in front of you, and as each thought comes up you imagine placing the thought on a leaf. As you visualize the thought on the leaf, you watch the leaf gently float down the stream–taking your thought with it. You do this with any and all thoughts that come up for you during this practice! Whether they're helpful or unhelpful thoughts, you practice this activity to strengthen your ability to CATCH your thoughts and then CHOOSE to let them go. This activity can be modified to imagine your thoughts on bubbles as they pop, appearing and disappearing into the clouds, or on cars passing by on the highway. Remember, each of these skills are simply suggestions and you are encouraged to get creative with ways that you can make them work for you!

CHANGE: Reframing Your Thoughts

One of the ways we can take some power away from unhelpful thoughts is by countering them with a more helpful thought. I'm not saying to take a thought that stings, like, *"I'm not good enough,"* and change it into a thought that is all full of sunshine and rainbows, like, *"I'm the BEST EVER!"* Such a drastic change would be difficult to pull off since you actually have to BELIEVE the new thought for it to have any kind of effect.

What you can do instead is change the thought into a more helpful one. This is where the growth mindset thinking comes into play! A simple way to make the thought more helpful is to add the phrase "...yet" after the thought. Watch what happens when we change the thought *"I'm not good enough"* to *"I'm not good enough, yet."* Doesn't it feel different?! It's not as heavy as it was before, and even includes a sprinkle of optimism in there too!

EMPOWER

CHOOSE: Allow yourself to take some time now to experiment with some of these skills! Try to pick a thought that only brings up slight discomfort to start with, and then notice how the intensity of the thought changes when you apply the different CHOOSE skills!

THOUGHT & INTENSITY (0-10)	CHOOSE SKILL	INTENSITY (0-10)

	Notice the thought	
	Slooooow it down	
	Speed it up	
	Silly voice	
	Sing it	
	Visualize letting go of the thoughts	

CHANGE: Remember, since this is a skill we are building, it is going to take some practice to get better over time at swapping out those pesky unhelpful thoughts for more helpful ones! Go ahead and give the CHANGE skill a shot with a common unhelpful thought that comes up for you:

ORIGINAL THOUGHT	CHANGE THOUGHT

MINDFULNESS

I wanted to take some time to introduce mindfulness and how it can be one of our most powerful tools with behavior change. A few years ago I would have rolled my eyes as soon as I saw the word "mindfulness," because I felt like one of the biggest skeptics out there! I was under the impression that mindfulness was about trying to embody the energy of a Buddhist monk, levitating on a mountain top, achieving total Nirvana, without a thought in his mind besides the word *Oooommmm*.

After doing some digging into the research, I discovered that it wasn't about trying to turn off your thoughts completely—which is what I believed at the time. It took me a while to get the hang of this mindfulness thaaaang, but with dedicated practice I started noticing the benefits of transforming my relationship with my thoughts and emotions, creating mini-miracles out of everyday moments, and being able to catch myself before lashing out at those who I care about.

Let's break down what mindfulness is and how it plays an important role in making lifestyle changes. Dr. Jon Kabat-Zinn, the founder and creator of the Mindfulness-Based Stress Reduction (MBSR) program, defines mindfulness as *"the awareness that arises from paying attention, on purpose, in the present moment and non-judgmentally."* There are some key aspects of that definition of mindfulness that play a starring role in our behavior change journey:

1. **Awareness**: We can't change what we don't know! So bringing awareness to the things we do that are holding us back will allow us to start making changes to help us move forward. Awareness is going to play a huge part throughout your transformation journey.
2. **Attention**: We need to pay attention to our actions and the impact they have on our well-being. Taking ourselves out of autopilot mode will help us to notice when we're

engaging in behaviors that are pulling us away from the life we desire.

3. **Purpose**: We want there to be purpose behind the actions we take, which means we need to be intentional about the choices we make.

4. **Present Moment**: It all starts with HERE and NOW—we can't go back and change the past, so focusing on what's happening in *this* moment gives us an opportunity to choose again.

5. **Non-judgmentally**: The more you can channel an attitude of curiosity instead of judgment, the stronger your forward momentum will build. Judging yourself (and others around you) creates a heaviness that will continue to weigh you down and hold you back from making progress.

In his TED Talk, Dr. Judson Brewer—who has some phenomenal books about habit change—discusses the benefits of incorporating curiosity when it comes to behavior change because curiosity is naturally rewarding for us humans! Here's where this REALLY comes in handy—when we develop habits, after encountering a cue in our habit loop we get URGES and CRAVINGS to engage in the behavior. This is that space we talked about earlier where we can make a CHOICE where we can disrupt and reprogram our Habit Loops!

This emphasizes the importance of our own ATTITUDE towards our lifestyle changes. Dr. Shauna Shapiro discusses how attitude plays a crucial role in mindfulness practices in her book, *Good Morning, I Love You*. In her own mindfulness journey, she is told a phrase by a monk at a meditation retreat that completely rocks her world—and I bet it will rock yours too!

"WHAT YOU PRACTICE GROWS STRONGER."

C'mon y'all...how freaking GOOD is that?! This is exactly what neuroplasticity is all about: strengthening our mental muscles. So what is it that YOU have been practicing when you've tried changing your habits before?

Impatience, frustration, self-judgment? Is that what you want to continue growing more of in your life? Eww, no way...I'm going to guess that just makes you feel like shit! So what is it that you would like to grow instead?

Patience, kindness, compassion? Mmmmm...yes PLEASE!

Let's take a look at how the seven attitudes of mindfulness can help us with changing our lives for the better...

- **Non-Judgment**: I know we've touched on this one quite a bit already, but it's worth repeating–judging yourself is not a successful route to sustainable change. Practice swapping out that judgment for curiosity and watch how different your journey feels.
- **Patience**: Listen, you are only just planting the seeds of change towards your desired life right now–you can't expect to harvest the fruits of your labor overnight! Remember to be patient with yourself and with the process, because these small steps you are taking will lead to your larger transformation over time.
- **Beginner's Mind**: How you can better tap into your curiosity is thinking about taking the perspective of a child– or maybe an alien–and viewing each of your experiences as if it were the first time you were giving it a go! This is helpful when you start trying new things to support your

change journey! Instead of thinking, *Oh this won't work for me*, without even trying it–open up to testing it out with curiosity and thinking, *Hmm...I wonder what this will teach me!* or *I wonder what I can learn from this!*

- **Non-Striving**: OK yes, we are setting goals throughout this journey–goals that we will be striving for! When it comes to practicing mindfulness and exploring new activities, we want to let go of any expectations around it. Think about it this way–if you decide to try a whole week of following a whole food, plant-based meal plan, try not to set any expectations around a desired outcome from this little experiment. If you focus too strongly on *I want to lose 5 pounds this week with this meal plan*–which is striving for a weight loss outcome–you might miss out on other magic taking place during this experiment! Basically, while we do want to set goals, we don't want to set expectations for the processes we engage in along the way. Fixating on the outcomes of these activities could throw us off track.

- **Trust**: You are your own best expert–that is why I can't tell you WHAT to do...because I'm not you! Part of this journey is learning how to trust yourself along the way as you begin exploring new skills and strategies for success in your lifestyle change journey.

- **Acceptance**: I'm going more in depth with this one in the next chapter, but you have to accept where you are starting and any uncomfortable emotions that come up along the way. The more we try to fight off those emotions, the stronger they will keep coming back. With acceptance, we learn to make room for those emotions to keep them from steering us off track when shit hits the fan in our lives.

- **Letting Go**: It's time to give yourself permission to let go of those stories you've been told or that you've told yourself over time that are holding you back or keeping you stuck from becoming the person you desire to be. You deserve to give yourself a break from the negative self-talk that has taken up space in your life for far too long. Letting go is an important step in moving forward. It will also be something you need to repeat over and over again, since those unhelpful thoughts and stories will show up frequently and try to keep you stuck. Practicing your skills to untangle yourself from those thoughts and stories your mind will bombard you with is part of letting go.

ENGAGE

Informal practices of mindfulness involve incorporating your full attention into different activities, like making coffee, showering, doing the dishes or mowing the lawn. It's about finding those ways to *really* engage your full attention and awareness into a present moment activity. Typically these practices are easier to start with than formal practice, so let's walk through an example together (*and if you're not a coffee drinker, maybe you won't appreciate this exercise much… but give it a try with something you enjoy!*):

Mindfully Drinking Coffee

If you're anything like me, you might brew your morning coffee cup or hit up the drive thru just so you can chug that glorious amount of caffeine to help flow through your veins as fast as humanly possible so you can perform and function during the day. But let's imagine for a moment that we slow down–it's a weekend morning, and you get to savor your morning coffee. From the moment you start making your morning coffee, your attention is focused on each and every detail of the process: the smell of the grounds as you open the container, the avalanche of the grounds as you scoop them into the filter, noticing the sound of the coffee maker turning on or the water heating, setting up your mug to catch each drop, watching the steam come out of the mug as it's brewed, the aroma gets stronger as it begins to fill the kitchen...and then maybe adding in your creamer and watching it dissolve into the coffee as the surface changes the color with the creamer mixed in. Then anticipating this delicious cup of coffee as you bring the mug up to your lips and the smell grows even stronger, feeling the warmth of the freshly brewed coffee spreading through the mug and into your hands...and then you take that first sip as you follow that sip passing from your mouth, into your esophagus, and aaaaaaaaall the way into your stomach...

WOW—did we just create a MAGICAL experience of drinking coffee?! I think we sure did! If you are not a coffee fan, you can try this with other beverages like tea, sparkling water, or even a glass of wine! Taking the time to mindfully enjoy your favorite beverage not only turns it into an experience, but it allows you to savor each and every sip you take instead of distractedly rushing through the drink without allowing yourself to enjoy it.

Informal mindfulness is about the mundane tasks we have in our lives that if we actually just pay attention to what we're doing it can take us out of our head, into the moment, and actually focus on engaging in the activity in front of us. Now some of you may actually be practicing mindfulness and task focused attention in different ways, because task focused attention is where you incorporate present moment awareness into the task at hand.

Formal mindfulness differs because these practices are structured, with specific amounts of time set aside to practice. Formal mindfulness is really where we're going to hit like the mental gym–that's where we're gonna get the most out of those mental repetitions! Whether you are sitting in silence or maybe listening to soft music while focusing on the breath or the body, the *practice* part of mindfulness comes in when we are catching the mind as it wanders and softly, gently inviting it back to the present moment with that compassionate, patient attitude. As you bring your attention back, instead of thinking, *Oh, I got distracted AGAIN, I totally suck at this mindfulness thing!!!* try to get playful with it and think *Hey! Come back here mind, you silly little brain you!* I will admit, getting mad at myself for being distracted is exactly how my mindfulness journey first started, but I was practicing frustration and irritation with myself–definitely NOT things I want to grow more of in my life! That just creates a whole bunch of ugly messiness.

Think of practicing mindfulness as your chance to build your mental muscles–it is what helps you catch your unhelpful thought and behavior patterns and empowers you to create space for change. There will be aspects of mindfulness that continue to show up throughout this book, especially when it comes to bringing awareness to our habits and working to change them.

Which CHOOSE and CHANGE skills did you find helpful?

What ways can you practice mindfulness in your own life?

Now that we've tackled some of the common challenges with mindset, let's talk about staying true to ourselves through...

Chapter 3:

Acceptance & Authenticity

You're allowed to sit in the suck…as long as you don't get stuck.

–Melyssa Allen

Sensitive Topic Warning
- *Body dysmorphia*
- *Eating disorders*

Just before I started writing this chapter, I had a crying spell in the shower, one on my boyfriend's shoulder, and another at my computer keyboard. The reason behind all the tears? I was trying out a new dance format and felt myself messing up the moves. As I compared myself to the hourglass body on the screen in front of me, moving effortlessly and shaking her hips and ass in ways I wish I could, my inner "mean girl" voice chimed in calling out all of my insecurities. And then the voice repeated all of the hurtful words I've heard over the years about my body... Sigh.

I've always loved to dance, but I also knew I would never make it into a career. I first got started dancing when I took ballet from third through sixth grade. During that time, I noticed that my body was bigger and fuller than the bodies of the other girls in class. I didn't see many other dancers who had the same shape as me. And the ones that did, weren't getting any of the starring roles in the shows—even though they were some of the strongest, most talented dancers I had ever seen.

Regardless of looking different, I didn't stop dancing. I remember how good I was too: I could keep the musical rhythm like nobody's business, and I was able to move my body gracefully. And while I wasn't quite as flexible as the other girls—and I still didn't *look* like a ballet dancer—my technique was solid. Eventually, I even learned to dance *en pointe*, which was one of my big goals for taking ballet in the first place. I dreamed of being able to twirl on my toes and looking as pretty and as strong as the other dancers. I wanted to be able to perform all those magical movements they did, too. So when I finally reached my goal, I was so sooooo happy. But all of my happiness came to a screeching halt one day after class.

I distinctly remember my ballet teacher, who also happened to be my grandma's best friend, walking past me one day and muttering something. I thought I heard her say, "I need you to stop and wait after class…." I was a little confused at the time, but I waited by her office door after all the other dancers in my class left like she'd asked me to. When she saw me, though, she walked over with a confused look on her face and said, "Melyssa, what are you still doing here?" And I replied, "I thought you asked me to wait…." To which she replied, "No, no, I told you that you need to **WATCH your weight!**"

I was in sixth grade.

And that is how insecurities, eating disorders, and body dysmorphia start, y'all…All it takes is some unintentional (or if you're dealing with a complete asshole, sometimes totally intentional) words. The words can crawl under your skin, creep deep into your heart, and get etched into your brain where they echo over and over and over again… And that is why I always recommend working with a therapist or counselor to take a deeper dive into how what you've been told or taught in the past is affecting you now. Because let me tell you… if you allow yourself to get all tangled up in the words that break you down, you may hold yourself back from the life you desire.

I am happy to say that, at the time, I was already considering leaving ballet to follow in my mom's athletic endeavors and pursue volleyball. When I got in the car after that class, I told her about wanting to quit ballet to play volleyball. To this day, I'm grateful that she didn't bombard me with questions about my decision that day. Instead, she just asked if I was sure that this was what I wanted and then supported me in making the change. I don't think

81

she knew why I decided to quit ballet until a few years ago. When we finally spoke about it, I remember talking about how, if I hadn't already been thinking about playing volleyball, my ballet instructor's hurtful words could have affected me in a much worse way.

The words we hear throughout our lifetime create stories we tell ourselves for years to come. It can be extremely hard to break out of old patterns of thinking, and depending on how deep-rooted those thoughts are, they can become ingrained beliefs about ourselves. And over time, as these types of self-deprecating thoughts and stories get repeated in our minds, they become a habit of how we think about ourselves.

Some of those words we hear could come from complete strangers, others from people who may even care about us. Regardless of where they come from, they can sting every time they pop back up from the depths of memories you try soooo hard to forget. And sometimes, the words we hear from someone else become so entangled in our minds that we can't tell the difference anymore between what we've been told and what we think about ourselves. I've had the–ahem–"pleasure" of having the following statements become recurring thoughts that turned into stories I told myself over time:

- "You're too fat to ever be a trainer at SeaWorld." -high school ex-boyfriend (*yup, a real winner there...*)
- "Hey, boobies!" -random guy at a bar (*totally original, bro...*)
- "You'd be able to dance better *en pointe* if you lost some weight. Plus, it would be easier on your toes if you weren't so heavy." –the entire ballet world

- "You'd be so much prettier if you just had a flatter stomach." -me to myself in the mirror (*thanks a lot, unrealistic societal standards*)

UGGGGHHHH... I don't know about you, but even reading those again made my stomach feel like it was falling out of my ass. So let's shift out of this painful walk down my memory lane and focus on applying what we've learned in the Mindset Matters chapter about taking power away from these hurtful little bastards (*AKA: our negative self-talk thoughts*). This is an important conversation because, chances are, you've used stories like these to bully yourself into changing your life, right?

And how did that go for you?

Maybe you were able to make some changes at first but, over time, slipped back into your familiar patterns and accepted defeat. After that, you probably found yourself in a flurry of self-critical thoughts that continued to hit you after you were already down.

Sound familiar, dear Change Maker?

EDUCATE

ACCEPTANCE

Wait... she wants me to do WHAT?! I didn't think I read the message from my friend, Kylie, the social media manager for a woman-owned small business called Not Only Pants (NOP), correctly. The message asked if I would be available to model NOP products at a photo shoot scheduled in Orlando. *Ummm... did she mean to send this message to somebody else? I'm not a model! This must be a mistake...*

I remained skeptical until Monica Delgado, the founder and creator of NOP, reached out to me. She explained how she wanted to include REAL bodies and promote more body diversity as part of her brand's mission! How freaking amazing was that?! But I still wasn't sure whether I wanted to put myself out there like that–standing in front of a camera only in my leggings and a sports bra...? SHEESH! Talk about an idea that sounded absolutely terrifying to me!

At the time, I was really working on my own self-love and self-acceptance, so agreeing to this opportunity would have been a GIANT step forward for me. Believe me when I tell you that, after I agreed to help them out, I immediately began thinking of any and every excuse in the book to cancel! I forgot I had a doctor's appointment... my car battery died... I had the shits from food poisoning... I got called into work! You name it, I considered it.

But then, I took a page out of Mel Robbins' book, *The 5 Second Rule*, and told myself I was excited, I was EXCITED! I kept repeating the words like a mantra to help keep my nerves at bay and try to convince my mind that my body's response was simply excitement–not gutwrenching terror or dread. Despite my attempts, though, as the photo shoot neared, I felt myself getting more and more self-conscious and regretting saying yes....

And when the day of the photo shoot finally arrived, all my negative thoughts and biggest insecurities were clamoring loudly for my attention. In fact, my mind was doing anything and everything to get me the fuck out of there and avoid vulnerability at all costs!!! But I didn't allow myself to get tangled up in those thoughts. Instead, I decided to use my skills of thinking about the thoughts differently.

At first, my mind continuously repeated that old story over and over again:
"I AM FAT–I'm the biggest one in the room! I AM SOOOO FAT."

Then, my compassionate self-talk spoke up to help me be brave and rise above my insecurities:

"Fat is something you HAVE, not something you ARE. You get the opportunity to be the body that you wish you had seen as a child growing up. You are not fat, you have fat–and so does everyone else on the planet!"

This change in my thinking was a HUUUUGE act of acceptance. Not only did I learn how to be with my body as it was, but also how to weather that storm of powerful emotions that tried to keep me from doing something scary! My acceptance made room for those emotions and thoughts and still allowed me to take action committed to my values. In this example, I was someone who did not *feel* completely confident in their body, but I chose to show up confidently with my body. I hope this story sticks with you as we work toward cultivating our inner cheerleader and drowning out that inner drill sergeant!

A lot of us think that being hard on ourselves, will give us the boost we need to make changes. But in reality, when we guilt and shame ourselves into trying to change, we only deactivate the learning centers in our brain! In her TED Talk, Dr. Shauna Shapiro does a wonderful job discussing how this self-judgemental approach prevents us from learning and growing. She also mentions that a patient and compassionate approach can help us learn from our shortcomings. The problem is we continue to default into our judgmental thought patterns because that is either what we learned through observation, what we were taught, or what we figured out on our own.

The solution to breaking through those patterns lies in choosing to relate to ourselves and our bodies differently. This topic could be an entire book in itself because it can be such a complicated process! In this book, however, we are only going to scratch the surface of ways to practice self-kindness and self-compassion. Keep those key themes in mind as you go forward–you will see them popping up over and over again.

Getting caught up in the comparison trap–and learning to be unsatisfied with your body unless it looks a certain way along the way–is the perfect combination for the emergence of body image issues. It is especially tough living in the day and age of the "highlight reel" on social media. Daily, we are bombarded by photos and videos edited or filtered to portray the people behind the screens looking their best. You want to know something wild?? There have been studies conducted that have discovered our brains interpret viewing a face that we KNOW is edited or filtered the same way as we would an unedited or unfiltered face. Regardless of the knowledge, the same parts of the brain are activated whether the face is real or fake, even though WE KNOW IT ISN'T REAL! Sheesh. No wonder social media can result in some serious struggles with our mental well-being.

The more we attempt to resist accepting our bodies as they are, in this moment, the tougher our change journey will be. Suppose you are continuously caught in the comparison trap of sizing up your body compared to all the other bodies you see in magazines, on social media, or in television shows and movies. In that case you are likely to become stuck or fall into an unhelpful downward spiral of negative thoughts and feelings.

When we fall into that downward spiral, we often experience self-sabotaging behaviors since the less positive we feel about ourselves, the less likely we are to do positive things for ourselves. And vice versa, the more positive we feel about ourselves, the more likely we are to engage in positive actions, which we will touch on in the next chapter. As humans, we tend to avoid discomfort as much as possible—if it doesn't feel good, we don't want it! This can lead us to try to escape, control, avoid, or numb our discomfort. Typically, we make these attempts through behaviors that provide us temporary relief from our uncomfortable experiences. These can include stress eating, trying to drink our problems away, scrolling through social media, etc.

In the last chapter, we discussed how to manage unhelpful thoughts more effectively—here, we are going to learn how to better manage our feelings! Remember, the only part of the Cognitive Triangle that we have control over is our behaviors. Therefore, when it comes to the thoughts and feelings that cause us discomfort, we need to learn new behaviors to deal with them instead of returning to those old, familiar patterns that take away from our health and well-being.

I like to think of our feelings and emotions as our family. There are some family members you are SO excited to see, and when they visit, you never want them to leave. That is typically how we feel about our positive emotions, like joy, love, and excitement. However, we also have those family members that show up uninvited, overstay their welcome, and are such a drag to be around, right? That is typically how we feel about our uncomfortable emotions, like grief, pain, and anger.

EMPOWER

How have you previously attempted to cope with uncomfortable emotions?

Think of a time when you were facing a challenge in life—what words of support and comfort from others did you find helpful?

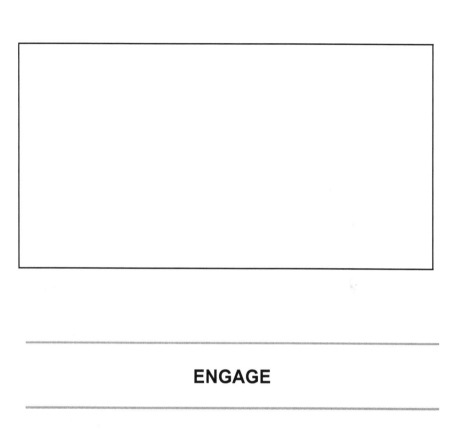

ENGAGE

You will likely fall off track and lose sight of your goals during this lifestyle-change journey. When that happens, it can be helpful to remind yourself of WHY you are putting in all that energy and effort to feel happier and healthier. The following practices are helpful in extending self-kindness and self-compassion to better manage uncomfortable emotions as they pop up! Here are some ways you can shift into a more supportive and patient path for change:

Self-Compassion Break: Notice how you're feeling (*"This hurts... This is stressful"*) and try naming your emotions. Are you feeling anger, fear, sadness, or something else altogether? Remember that pain is part of life and every human experiences it *("I'm not alone... Other people feel this way... We all struggle in life")*. Place one or both hands over where you notice your emotional pain, and do your best to extend kindness toward your pain and yourself. Maybe even ask, *"What do I need to hear right now to express kindness towards myself?"* See if there is a phrase that comforts you (*"May I be strong... May I forgive myself... May I accept myself as I am"*).

Supportive Touch: Place one or both hands over your heart. If that feels too vulnerable, maybe try placing your hands on your thighs, over your stomach, or the opposite elbows. Feel where your hands connect to the rest of your body. Take two to three intentional, deep breaths. Notice your body moving as you breathe. Maybe pair your breathing with a phrase, *"Inhale kindness, exhale judgment... Inhale compassion, exhale criticism... Inhale confidence, exhale doubt...."*

Soften, Soothe, Allow:
Soften your body: Take a deep breath and try to release areas of tension or tightness. *Soothe yourself:* Think of comforting phrases or practice supportive touch. *Allow your experience to just be:* Instead of trying to fight off uncomfortable emotions, try to see if you can make space for them instead to help them pass by more quickly.

Think of a Friend or Loved One: Take a moment to imagine a friend or loved one coming to you expressing similar challenges that you are facing. What would you say to help comfort and support them? Once you think about what you would say to them, see if you can practice extending those same words of comfort and support toward yourself.

EDUCATE

AUTHENTICITY

I know sometimes we might wish we could do things differently. Personally, I wish I could finish everything I've started! But I get distracted by "Shiny Object Syndrome" and move on to new things before following through with existing projects—which is likely why I could never complete a full fitness and nutrition program! Now, if I continuously put up resistance around accepting that is a behavior pattern of mine, I would never allow myself the chance to explore opportunities to find what works best for ME.

There have been so many times in my life that I've seen people doing things a certain way and thinking to myself, *"Jeez Melyssa, why can't you just get your shit together and do what they did?!"* I'd want to try all these fitness and nutrition plans that showed people getting amazing results, but when I actually had to follow through, I'd get bored, feel restricted from foods I enjoyed, and develop unhealthy relationships with both food and exercise. For a while, I would be obsessed with tracking my calories and rigidly fixed on not going over my daily "allowance" of calories. I would force myself to do the workouts, even though I was DREADING them all day... but I had to follow the plan. In the end, these "healthy lifestyle" programs would cause me so much stress, they'd result in disordered eating behaviors. Actually, I would often *gain* weight even as I was trying so desperately to lose it!

The structured fitness and nutrition plans work extremely well for some people, and I kept wishing that I could be one of those people! But they just wouldn't work for me, no matter how hard I tried. The more resistance I put up around that realization, the more I found it difficult to find the motivation and desire to keep trying to change.

It wasn't until I learned to accept the me that is *me*, here and now, that I was able to start actually exploring strategies that worked for me and made it–dare I say–*easier* to follow through with actions that supported my health and well-being. Please realize the more you struggle against who you are and how you "BE" in the world, the more difficulties you will face in taking actions to support your desired future self.

EMPOWER

How would you, unapologetically, describe your authentic self? The you that is you–right here, right now?

EDUCATE

That realization is where authenticity comes into play. Accepting yourself for who you are is the key to change, so you can stop fighting to change yourself and learn how to work with yourself along the way.

I remember never feeling like I fully "fit in" anywhere—I didn't have friend groups, and even in my extracurricular activities like volleyball and orchestra, I just never felt like I really "clicked" with anyone. Over time, I began to adapt how I acted to make myself feel like I fit in. I started taming my inner weird kid, pretending I didn't think dolphins were *that* cool, and rehearsing things in my head before I said them out loud, so I didn't sound like an idiot. All of that was A LOT of work. Hiding my true self resulted in surface-level friendships as I thought I needed to find a group to fit in with rather than having genuine connections that could evolve into a group of their own!

After I graduated from college, I continued this pattern. At one point, I joined the Disney's Animal Program as an Aquatic Research intern. One day, during a team building exercise, the entire research department took part in the StrengthsFinder assessment.. The results showed my top two strengths were Positivity and WOO (Winning Others Over). My strengths, along with those of the nearly 50 other team members, were included in a slideshow presented at our department meeting. Guess how

many people had Positivity and WOO in their top five...? Yep–
JUST ME. Oh, the *HUMANITY*. I felt completely called out among
a group of scholars for being the girl with her head in the clouds,
dreaming of playing with marine mammals someday. I tried to own
it at the time, but I felt somewhat ashamed that I didn't have
strengths like Analytical or Detail-Oriented. How was I ever going
to make it as a respected individual among the scientific
community?!

For the longest time after that, I kept trying to prove my "worth" by
attempting to suppress my true, unabashedly positive self to fit in
the metaphorical box of what is "expected" from society. I
dedicated so much time and energy to strengthening what I
viewed as my weaknesses at the time.. Since I also wanted to "fit
in" with others, whether that was in my doctoral program or my
corporate role at the hospital, I worked hard to dress and act the
part I was *supposed* to play. In fact, I worked so hard that I began
losing the best parts of myself.

It wasn't until I truly began working on rediscovering who I was,
outside of those groups I was trying to force myself into, that I
found freedom in accepting and embracing who I was. I now
utilize my strength of Positivity and my WOO factor to help inspire
and motivate others to change their lives while working to change
my own as well.

The longer that YOU, dear Change Maker, attempt to hide your
true self, fit yourself into a box, and try to follow what everyone
else is doing, the more off-course you might get. Instead, embrace
and accept yourself as you are, learn to play to your strengths,
and find what works best for YOU. That newfound knowledge will

guide you toward your desired future self and allow for a much smoother path along the way.

Engaging in the process of self-exploration is likely one of the most helpful things you can do for yourself as you embark on this lifestyle-change journey. There are parts of you that only want to support you and cheer you on through your lifestyle-change journey. And there are also parts of you that are scared of failing and will try to hold you back. Those are the parts of yourself that you want to accept and ask to tag along for the ride. Trying to fight them off and inadvertently letting them steer you in the opposite direction of your goals will only exhaust you.

So please take some time now to allow yourself to release whatever expectations you have of how your lifestyle-change journey "should" look, whether they are based on what the world has told you or your self-imposed beliefs. Let that shit goooooo, and let's get ready to roll with *your unapologetically authentic badass self who is ready to do the damn thing!*

I want you to belt out *THIS IS ME* like Keala Settle from the movie, *The Greatest Showman*! Drop a good ole *DAMN, IT FEELS GOOD TO BE ME* like Andy Grammer sings in his anthem for authenticity! Find your own version of a reminder to yourself of your uniqueness to make sure you stay true to *you*.

Take some time to answer the questions below, keeping in mind how your answers may affect your journey to lasting behavior change.

EMPOWER

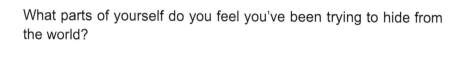

What parts of yourself do you feel you've been trying to hide from the world?

What are you afraid would happen if you let the world see those parts?

What are some of your best qualities as a person? What do you think your "superpower" is when it comes to your strengths?

Staying true to your authentic self, on a scale of one (slow and steady) to ten (challenging myself), with how much intensity do you want to approach your lifestyle-change journey?

If you answered toward the higher end of the scale, what are some ways you can manage your "inner critic" voice when you slip up on your lifestyle change-journey? What are some of the ways you can shift out of a space of bullying yourself to supporting yourself instead?

ENGAGE

Letter to Yourself: In this activity, I would like you to imagine a past version of yourself–a version of you that was trying so very hard to change your life for the better. This past version of yourself has temporarily veered off course from your desired Life Map. Now, I want you to imagine that past version of yourself sitting across from you, at the exact moment when you decided to give up on trying to make positive changes for yourself. You can see this past version of yourself is disappointed, defeated, frustrated....

What do you wish this past version of you could have heard to keep going? What words of kindness, comfort, and support would you offer to that same version of yourself sitting across from you now? Take some time and give yourself permission to be vulnerable. If you need to take a break during this activity, please do so.

Keep this letter to yourself somewhere where you can access it easily whenever you need those words of encouragement to help guide and support you on your journey.

To continue this positive path toward healthy lifestyle changes, we're now going to explore the fields of...

Chapter 4:

Positive Health & Lifestyle Medicine

"If we could give every individual the right amount of nourishment and exercise, not too little and not too much, we would have found the safest way to health."

– Hippocrates

In the previous chapter, we began exploring some of the aspects of positive psychology, which is the focus of this chapter. More and more research is demonstrating the reciprocal and reinforcing link between positive experiences and healthy lifestyle behaviors. This is an important framework to explore because we're living in a time where mental wellness struggles are more prevalent than ever.

Not to be a bummer Change Makers... but recent research has shown that six out of ten people in the US are diagnosed with one or more chronic diseases, like obesity, type 2 diabetes, hypertension, cardiovascular disease, and even certain types of cancers. But did you know that up to 80% of lifestyle-related chronic diseases could be prevented, treated, or reversed by changing how we live? Even considering genetics, modifying our behaviors is the most effective way to reduce our risk of lifestyle-related chronic diseases!

You might not know this, but you have the ability to change the trajectory of your family history in certain cases. You might be thinking, *"Oh, well, heart disease runs in my family, so it's only a matter of time before it gets me too."* Guess what, though? We now know that your family health history is not necessarily YOUR destiny, thanks to the study of epigenetics!

Epigenetics is defined by the Center for Disease Control (CDC) as the study of how your behaviors and the environment you're in can affect the way your genes work. DAMN! How cool is THAT? We can actually modify the way our bodies interpret certain DNA sequences based on our lifestyle choices. I don't know about you, but I totally geek out over learning stuff like that!

So listen, y'all, just because you have a family history of certain chronic diseases doesn't mean you are destined to follow the same path! Yes, your genetics have a certain effect over your susceptibility and predisposition to developing lifestyle-related chronic diseases, but your health journey isn't set in stone.

Besides genetic information, do you know what else we tend to inherit from our families…?

That's right–our lifestyle behaviors! And as previous chapters have mentioned, lifestyle behaviors are learned behaviors, which means they can be changed! YOU have the power to change the trajectory of your own health by creating and following positive health habits.

Isn't that great news?!

Despite the great news, though, a movement towards positive health is needed now more than ever. For the first time in human history, our projected lifespan is on the decline. If you're considered a "millenial"–I'm talking to my people in our 30s and 40s–we're projected to have a shorter expected lifespans than our parents! And even though we live in an era with the most advanced technological capabilities, predictions of lifespan for the upcoming generations are even shorter.

Unfortunately, the biggest reason for these predictions is the way we're living. The combination of factors, like ridiculously processed foods, sitting for endless hours throughout the day, getting sucked into our screens, and living in a world that is more stressed out and sleep deprived than EVER, there has been an alarmingly rapid rise in lifestyle-related chronic diseases. I don't mean to say all that to make it sound like our future is full of doom-and-gloom, but it is helpful for us to recognize the things we do have control over to give us the best chance at a long, healthy life.

There are certain parts of the world called the Blue Zones, where the populations have the highest concentration of centenarians (*people who live to be 100+ years old!*). In these Blue Zones, researchers have discovered common lifestyle and environmental factors that support health and well-being that are now referred to as the Power 9®:

1. **Move naturally**: Relying on walking as the main mode of transportation means many Blue Zone communities are naturally more active due to the environments they live in.
2. **Purpose:** Staying connected to what is most meaningful and having a sense of purpose leads to greater longevity.
3. **Downshift**: Taking time to rest each day aids in recovery from life stressors.
4. **80% rule:** Instead of overindulging, these cultures follow the guideline of eating until you are around 80% full.
5. **Plant slant:** The dietary lifestyles in the Blue Zones are more plant-based, with an average consumption of animal products at a small serving of three to four ounces about five times per month.
6. **Wine at 5:** Studies of the Blue Zones have found that enjoying a glass or two of wine at dinner with friends or family can be beneficial. Ironically, we will discuss the health risks of alcohol consumption in an upcoming chapter. The reason why the Wine at 5 guideline works for the Blue Zone cultures is that they don't engage in binge drinking behaviors.

7. **Belong:** Being part of a community has been linked to increased life expectancy. Regardless of whether it is a spiritual community or not, a sense of belonging contributes to feeling part of something bigger than yourself.
8. **Loved ones first:** Keeping close family ties and having a life partner support all aspects of well-being.
9. **Right tribe:** Having strong social support is linked to numerous positive health benefits and favorable health behavior changes.

We can already see how the Blue Zones framework encompasses different aspects of lifestyle medicine and positive psychology together. Remember, though, if you're anything like me and reading this list made you feel terrified because you don't practice many of these habits, it's not too late to make a change!

EDUCATE

LIFESTYLE MEDICINE

The field of lifestyle medicine has been EXPLODING because we are living in a world where the healthy choice isn't always the easy choice. Not to mention our healthcare system operates more like a "sick-care" system when it treats the symptoms of lifestyle-related chronic diseases through overmedication instead of addressing the root cause of the diseases. When you need medications to treat the symptoms of your medications to treat the symptoms of your illness–there's GOT to be a better way to do things! Don't take this to mean that I'm anti-medication–that's absolutely not the case! Medications have their place in treatment plans. The problem we face, however, is the OVER prescription of pharmaceuticals for health challenges that could be supported by, or even resolved through, lifestyle prescriptions.

That's where lifestyle medicine comes in. This branch of medicine helps us focus on reducing behaviors that put our health at risk for chronic diseases and replacing them with health-promoting habits. Lifestyle medicine is defined as "the use of evidence-based lifestyle interventions as a primary modality to prevent, treat and often reverse chronic disease." The six pillars of lifestyle medicine include:

- A whole-food, plant-predominant eating pattern
- Regular physical activity
- Restorative sleep
- Effective stress management
- Avoidance of risky substances, like tobacco, vaping, and alcohol
- Positive social connections.

These six lifestyle behaviors have been demonstrated over and over again in the research to have the strongest predictors of quality of life and longevity. The idea of lifestyle medicine isn't anything new, of course. We know we should be exercising, eating healthy, sleeping well, and stressing less. Still, there is a massive disconnect between knowing we SHOULD do these things and actually DOING them. This is typically referred to as the "intention-behavior gap" because, while we might have every good intention to change, actually following through on the behavior change is MUCH harder! So lifestyle medicine now uses prescribed therapeutic lifestyle interventions to address those pesky behavioral risk factors we are so inclined to develop!

The American College of Lifestyle Medicine (ACLM) formally introduced the field of lifestyle medicine in 2004, although the concepts of behavioral risk reduction have been around MUCH longer than that! Although the ideas behind healthy lifestyle behaviors have been around for ages–even during the times of Hippocrates!–training programs have not included information on prescribing lifestyle changes until recently. That has been a large problem with the current healthcare system (*at least in the United States*) is that clinicians, like doctors and nurses, aren't extensively taught how to coach patients effectively through behavior change. While our healthcare providers can tell us WHAT we need to do, they don't necessarily tell us HOW to do it. And figuring it out on our own can be extremely overwhelming!

The structure of healthcare visits and insufficient insurance coverage are other complicating factors in our broken healthcare system. Honestly y'all, how in the world are clinicians supposed to have meaningful conversations with patients about behavior changes when they are limited to 15-minute encounters?! *Spoiler alert:* With all the information clinicians are required to collect during visits, it is EXTREMELY difficult for them to navigate conversations promoting effective behavior change, although it is not impossible.

To fill these large gaps in patient care, health and well-being coaches have emerged to help guide and support patients on their behavior change journeys! As I've mentioned in the introduction, coaches don't tell you what you need to do; rather, they work with you as a team to co-create your goals toward change. So, while I will be sharing information with you in this book based on my training as a health and well-being coach, it is up to YOU to actually put in the work to make change happen in your life!

You know that cliche, "Knowledge is power"? I hate to break it to you, but that is total bullshit! If you don't do anything with the knowledge you gain, how is that going to be helpful at all?! Instead, the phrase should say, "APPLIED knowledge is power," because you actually have to practice what you learn to get any of the benefits of knowing the information!

At the risk of sounding all doomy-and-gloomy again, I need to point out that we are currently living through a public health crisis and I'm not even referring to the COVID-19 pandemic that continues to rear its ugly head even as I write this chapter. We are living in a time when lifestyle-related chronic diseases are running rampant and leading to significant declines in physical, mental, and emotional well-being. Now, more than ever, we are being called to take a more proactive role in our health and well-being. We CAN take action to protect ourselves from following a similar path that our family members who live with chronic diseases are walking on.

The first step in your change journey is acknowledging that you want to take action and make choices that support your well-being. The next step is evaluating what you need to do to move toward your healthiest, happiest self. The final step is figuring out the "how" that will work best for you and then developing systems of support, accountability, and commitment to be the driving force behind your desire to change.

POSITIVE HEALTH

Taking this desire for public health promotion even one step further, the emergence of the positive health movement is another valuable addition to the healthcare world. Dr. Martin Seligman, considered to be the father of Positive Psychology, defines positive health as the scientific study of "health assets." These health assets serve as protective factors against illnesses and negative health outcomes, while also contributing to an increased sense of well-being. I love the basis of the positive health movement because it shifts the health paradigm from an absence of illness to an actual state of optimal health and a sense of thriving!

Research has begun examining the link between lifestyle medicine and positive psychology in behavior change. Positive psychology studies the strengths that enable people and communities to thrive and plays an integral role in positive health. Dr. Barbara Frederickson and her team proposed the model of the upward spiral theory of lifestyle change, where positive emotions and positive health behaviors demonstrate a reciprocal, reinforcing relationship. When we participate in behaviors that support our health, we experience positive affect. Likewise, when we experience positive affect, we are more inclined to make choices supportive of our health and well-being.

Research exploring positive psychology practices has demonstrated well-being benefits such as enhanced mood, improved physical health, and increased longevity. Basically, positive psychology boils down to helping people with feeling

WELL versus just feeling "better" or "OK." Let's be clear, though, positive psychology is completely different from the toxic positivity you may see sprinkled in throughout our society with phrases like, like "*Just be positive! It will all be fine. Everything happens for a reason, just think happy thoughts! It could always be worse.*"

EWWW...OK, I know I've been guilty of repeating these phrases at times, but I've done my best to stop saying them when I realized how dismissive they are of our experiences during life's challenges. Positive psychology differs from toxic positivity because it doesn't try to ignore or gloss over your challenges. Rather, positive psychology empowers you to take action that gives your well-being a boost, while honoring the struggles and challenges you may be facing.

Instead of bullying yourself into changing, can you be open to learning how to become your own best cheerleader for a change? Being able to support ourselves on this journey creates that sustainable change we all desire!

Explore your strengths: So often, we focus on getting better at what we suck at that we miss the opportunity to take advantage of what we're already GOOD at! Playing to our strengths can be massively helpful in propelling us forward in our lifestyle-change journey! If you haven't taken the time to explore your strengths, there are some wonderful tools like the Values In Action (VIA) Character Strengths Survey to help you identify your personal strengths. You might also find it helpful to reflect on times in your life when things were going well. You could use that information to help you explore what strengths you demonstrated during those times and how they could be useful to you now!

Treat laughter as medicine: When you're feeling "stuck in the suck," try turning to laughter to help you bust out of that funk! Engaging in laughter is also great for our health, even when it isn't genuine! You know the phrase, *"fake it 'til you make it"*? Well, laughter (and smiling!) fits that sentiment perfectly because forcing yourself to laugh or smile, tricks your brain into releasing happy hormones and neurotransmitters. So even if you're pretending, you still get the physiological benefits of laughing! Pretty cool life hack, huh?!

Use the PERMA Model: PERMA is an acronym that breaks down to: **P**ositive emotions, **E**ngagement (a state of flow), **R**elationships, **M**eaning, and **A**ccomplishment. This model provides a framework for enhancing well-being through participating in activities that correspond with its elements. For instance, to experience positive emotions, do things that give you a mood boost! The engagement part of the acronym isn't the *"you shoulda put a ring on it"* kind. Instead, engagement refers to being fully engaged in an activity that you enjoy to the point that the time just FLIES by! We also want to have a solid support system to turn to and continue to foster positive relationships in our lives. Activities that are meaningful to you or give you a sense of purpose lead to feelings of connectedness to your values. Experiencing a sense of accomplishment–no matter how small–can help us to stay motivated and give us a confidence boost!

Find activities that incorporate all the elements to take advantage of the benefits of PERMA. For example, teaching group fitness classes checks ALL the boxes of PERMA for me. I get a burst of positive emotions while teaching, I find myself in a state of flow where the time flies by, I'm forming relationships with the people in my classes, I find making fitness FUN meaningful, and I am left with a sense of accomplishment once the class finishes! While it's helpful to find activities that align with all of the elements, even activities that fit with one of them can be beneficial! Here are some reflection prompts to help guide you in finding activities that maximize PERMA:

- **P:** What can you do to increase positive emotions in yourself? What are some of your go-to mood boosters?
- **E:** What "flow" activities can you do regularly?
- **R:** What relationships can add positivity to your life? What can you do to increase positive interactions?
- **M:** What activities are meaningful to you and how can you include them in your professional and personal life?
- **A:** What goals can you pursue that align with your values and passions and that you can achieve successfully?

Gratitude: Gratitude is often defined as "the quality of being thankful," which can be a powerful tool for our well-being. While we can't stop ourselves from feeling certain emotions, gratitude is a way to help us refocus our attention from what is burdening our lives to what is blessing our lives. Research has demonstrated that actively engaging in a gratitude practice can lead to greater enthusiasm, energy, and empowerment to offer help to others.

The power of gratitude is absolutely incredible—it can help you shift out of a funky space and bring things back into perspective. My absolute FAVORITE musician of all time, Andy Grammer, created this mind blowing song collaboration with Fitz & the Tantrums called "The Wrong Party." The message of the song is that we're missing out on this grand ole party called life, while we're at "the wrong party" chasing all these elusive things, attempting to impress other people, and stressing over the little things! (*Seriously Andy, HUGE fan of your music and love everything you do!*) Learning how to shift from focusing on our burdens to focusing on our blessings, can be one of our greatest human superpowers!

Here are some simple gratitude practices to try out:

- **Gratitude Journaling**: Set aside some time to journal about three specific things that you are grateful each day! Try to find something unique each and every day and try not to repeat any of the things you are thankful for for at least a week. My personal practice includes these three prompts: 1) Today I am grateful for...; 2) I am looking forward to...; 3) My favorite part of today was....

- **Gratitude Check-in**: Take a few seconds to bring to mind something that makes you smile or someone you love. Think about that thing or person in as much detail as you can for a brief moment during your day and notice how you feel after this practice! You can also use this as a family activity at the dinner table.

- **Gratitude Compliment**: Share some kind words with someone in your life and tell them why you are grateful to have them in your life!

EMPOWER

ACTIVITY: On average, how much physical activity do you participate in during the week?

NUTRITION: On average, how many servings of fruits and vegetables per day do you consume?

SLEEP: On average, how many hours of sleep do you get per night?

STRESS: How effectively do you feel you manage the stress in your daily life?

SUBSTANCE USE: Do you smoke/vape/drink alcohol? If so, how much and how often?

SOCIAL: Overall, how connected to others in your life do you feel?

ENGAGE

Mel Robbins has a section in her book, "The High 5 Habit," that talks about self-acceptance and how our relationship with our bodies affects our ability to change. She mentions how we can't hate our bodies and love ourselves at the same time—OOF! That's such a true statement. We really need to take a moment to step back and reflect on how our bodies have supported us over our lifetime.

So, in this practice, I invite you to write a letter of gratitude to your body. I would like you to thank your body for all the things it does for you on a daily basis, especially those that often get overlooked when we're picking ourselves apart in the mirror. Just like in our previous practice of writing a letter to ourselves, if you need to take a break during this activity, please do so.

Here are some optional prompts for you if you're having trouble getting started:
How has your body helped you throughout your lifetime? What daily miracles does your body gift you with that you don't even have to think about? What are some compliments you have received in the past, and how can you extend those same compliments toward yourself? What words of kindness does your body crave to hear?

I want to take a quick moment now to debrief and ask how you felt about completing that activity?? If you skipped it, I totally get it. Maybe you didn't feel like you were in the right headspace to get vulnerable with yourself right now, but please make sure you revisit it. This activity can be a helpful tool to shift out of a negative space. It can also give you a boost of positive emotions that can lead to more positive choices throughout the day!

In the next few chapters, we will be reviewing the six pillars of lifestyle medicine for health and well-being as well as the guidelines for optimal health. Even if you think you know all about a particular topic, I would encourage you to still read the chapters with that open-minded curiosity we discussed earlier and engage with the activities along the way to continue learning and exploring this valuable information!

Let's get started with our first–and I might argue our most important–pillar of lifestyle medicine and learn how we can better...

Chapter 5:

Invest in Your Rest

"My mother told me to follow my dreams…
so I took a nap!"

–Unknown

Choose the statement that best reflects your current feelings about your sleep health…

- I don't need to make changes with my sleep habits.
- I can't make changes with my sleep habits.
- I might need to make changes with my sleep habits.
- I will make changes with my sleep habits.
- I am making changes with my sleep habits.

Regardless of which option you chose above Change Makers, please don't skip out on this section! You never know what you could learn that might support your lifestyle change journey!

EDUCATE

Fun facts about sleep…
- Did you know that we can survive longer without food and water than without SLEEP?!
- Did you know that driving while drowsy can be just as, if not more, dangerous than driving buzzed or drunk?!?
- Did you know that getting the recommended amount of sleep each night can help prevent wrinkles?! I meeean, hello, gorgeous skin! It's called beauty sleep for a reason y'all!

My passion for teaching about healthy sleep habits began during my clinical internship for my master's program. I had the pleasure of working with Dr. Diane Robinson's team at the Integrative Medicine Department, which also housed the local Cancer Support Community. During this internship, I was included as a researcher in a study examining a telephone-delivered Cognitive-

Behavioral Therapy for Insomnia (CBTi) program for cancer patients and survivors. This experience helped me realize just how important sleep was.

As you will learn in the following few paragraphs, everyone can benefit from better sleep. However, as you can imagine, restful sleep and addressing sleep difficulties is even more critical for the population undergoing cancer treatment and cancer survivors. I am not exaggerating when I say the experience I had facilitating these CBTi sessions was a COMPLETE game changer for me! I worked with cancer patients and survivors to transform their unhelpful thoughts and behaviors around their sleep patterns into more helpful ones, and saw some phenomenal outcomes for the study participants!!! You might wonder, "*How in the WORLD do our thoughts and behaviors affect our sleep?!*" Well, just hang tight because we will definitely be talking about that soon, and YOU, too,might experience a total transformation in your sleep habits!

Sleep is probably the most important thing we can do for our physical, mental, and emotional well-being. And yet, it is usually the first thing we sacrifice when we are "busy" in our lives. But we need to continue prioritizing restful, restorative sleep! Why is that? Sleep is the "reset button" for our brains and bodies. Recommended amounts of restorative sleep help us to purge the toxins that build up during the day from our brains and our bodies. In addition, sleep resets and renews our energetic resources to support us in functioning at our best throughout the day. Sleep is the equivalent of plugging in your phone at night–you need the appropriate amount of time to recharge your own batteries!

You may be thinking, "*I just don't NEED that much sleep. I can function fine on only four to five hours per night....*" I'm going to call bullshit on that one! Maybe you were raised thinking that the less you slept, the more dedicated you were to your work/family/etc., but the problem with that line of thinking is that maaaaay be true in the short term...but in the long run? That kind of chronic sleep deprivation can have some seriously negative impacts on your health and even shorten your lifespan! You know that old cliche, "*I'll sleep when I'm dead?*" Welp! That latter part may come sooner than you'd like if you are not prioritizing sleep now!

Don't worry; we're not going to dig too deep into the super science-y stuff here. However, as you start to understand how sleep affects our bodies and brains, I hope you will let go of the unhelpful stories you may have developed around your sleep patterns. I also invite you to begin prioritizing sleep as one of your top self-care strategies and to open up to a healthier way of allowing your whole self to rest and recharge. Your entire person—and your wellness—are affected by your sleep health, so if you feel like you're not getting the most out of your sleep, keep reading. I'm about to rock your world with some ways that you can get better rest to feel your absolute BEST!

I'm not exaggerating. LITERALLY, every system and function of your body and brain will perform better with restful, restorative sleep. That means you'll have better digestion, a stronger immune system, a healthier heart, better memory recall, faster reaction times, and gorgeous skin with fewer wrinkles. And did I mention increased desires…if you know what I mean (*wink wink*)… and better performance in the sheets, too? I meeeean…who wouldn't want that?!

Unfortunately, that means when we are sleep deprived, we experience negative impacts on nearly every system in our bodies and the functioning of our brains! It's essential to recognize how not getting enough sleep affects our mental, physical, emotional, and social well-being. Let's take some time to reflect on your current sleep habits.

EMPOWER

Recommended Sleep Guidelines

While we are all unique individual human beings, there are general recommendations for sleep duration. Regardless of age, the recommended sleep needed is at least seven hours per night, according to organizations like the National Institutes of Health and the National Sleep Foundation (NSF). Here are the sleep recommendations from the NSF based on age:

AGE	SLEEP NEEDED
Birth - 2 months	12 - 18 hours
3 - 11 months	14 - 15 hours
1 - 3 years	12 - 14 hours
2 - 5 years	11 - 13 hours
5 - 10 years	10 - 11 hours
10 - 17 years	8.5 - 9.5 hours
17 or older	7 - 9 hours

I want us to pause here. Think about how you feel about your sleep and rate each question on a scale of zero to ten...

Do you feel you get enough sleep based on the recommended seven to nine hours per night guideline?

(*definitely not*) 0 - 1 - 2 - 3 - 4 - 5 - 6 - 7 - 8 - 9 - 10 (*absolutely!*)

How refreshed do you typically feel in the morning when you wake up?

(*still exhausted*) 0 - 1 - 2 - 3 - 4 - 5 - 6 - 7 - 8 - 9 - 10 (*ready for the day!*)

How many hours per sleep (on average) are you getting each night?

How much time (on average) are you spending in bed each night?

If you don't know how much time you spend in bed and how long you're asleep, that's okay! Towards the end of this section, there is an optional sleep log that you can use to track your sleep patterns and build greater awareness of your sleep habits.

EDUCATE

It's important to take some time to get a basic understanding of sleep health so that you can begin connecting the dots on how your lifestyle choices affect your sleep patterns. Remember, this knowledge may seem boring or not helpful initially, but understanding the processes can often help us recognize where we can make some changes!

Sleep Cycles

There are four stages of sleep, and they consist of two main blocks: Non-Rapid Eye Movement (NREM, Stages 1-3) and Rapid Eye Movement (REM).

Stage 1: This is the lightest stage of sleep, sometimes referred to as "drifting off," where your eye movement and muscle activity begin to slow down as you start to relax. If you've ever had that feeling of falling that caused you to jerk awake, you experienced it in this light stage of sleep!

Stage 2: This is the intermediate stage of sleep that prepares for a deeper sleep. The brain waves become slower, and your heart rate and body temperature drop. This is your slow and steady entrance into deep sleep.

Stages 3 & 4: In these deep sleep stages, the final ones in the Non-REM (non-rapid eye movement) sleep sequence, your body and brain slow down even more. This type of sleep helps to restore energetic resources, repair muscle tissue, strengthen bones, and support immune functioning.

REM: This is the deep sleep where activity in the brain and body actually increases. While in this stage, your heart rate and blood pressure rise, breathing becomes quicker, dreaming takes place, and your eyes move back and forth rapidly (hence, REM: rapid eye movement). Meanwhile, your limbs and major muscle groups act as if they are temporarily paralyzed. SO weird, right?! In this stage, your brain consolidates and processes the events from the previous day to store them in your memory bank.

An average sleep cycle lasts around 90-110 minutes.

- You may notice increased drowsiness the next day if your sleep cycle is disrupted during the night.
- This is also why "snoozing" becomes a problem. As you hit the snooze button, you jolt yourself out of your lightest stage of sleep (stage 1). This rude awakening causes you to feel sleepier throughout the day due to a phenomenon referred to as "sleep inertia!" Moral of the story: *lose the snooze!* I'm going to plug Mel Robbins' book *The 5 Second Rule* here. In her work, Mel does a PHENOMENAL job explaining how choosing to snooze was impacting every part of her life and how it changed once she started getting out of bed right away. The book is such a great read!

"Sleep Busters"

Certain things can interfere with our sleep, but we can work towards changing them or working around them. I like to call these our "*Sleep Busters.*" We want to swap them out for "*Sleep Boosters*" that will promote healthy sleep!

Check off which of these Sleep Busters you currently experience or engage in:

- Unhelpful thoughts
- Staying in bed when you can't sleep
- Doing other activities in bed, like reading, watching TV, worrying, etc.
- Snoring (yourself or your partner)
- Pets
- Kids
- Drinking Alcohol
- Drinking Caffeine
- Heavy meals before bed
- Screen time
- Stress & worry
- Uncomfortable bedroom environment
- Ambient light and noise
- Trying to force yourself to go to sleep
- Nightmares
- Pain
- Chronic illness
- Sleep disorders
  - *Restless Leg Syndrome*
  - *Insomnia*
  - *Sleep Apnea*
  - *DISCLAIMER: I know I had a disclaimer at the beginning of this book, but I just want to emphasize that you should always consult your primary care provider or a sleep specialist to rule out any underlying medical conditions that could be contributing to your sleep health. The information I present in this book is strictly educational and should not be taken as medical advice or diagnosis.*

This list is a brief overview, but you will learn more about how these interfere with sleep when you read about "Sleep Boosters!"

EMPOWER

Chronic sleep deprivation is linked to MANY negative health consequences, which you can find listed below (*keep in mind, this is not an exhaustive list*).

PHYSICAL	weakened immune system weight gain slower healing of the body skin wrinkles increased inflammation impaired sexual performance increased risk of… <ul><li>heart attack</li><li>heart failure</li><li>stroke</li><li>high blood pressure</li><li>obesity</li><li>type 2 diabetes</li><li>certain cancers</li><li>falls due to impaired balance</li></ul>
MENTAL AND/OR EMOTIONAL	increased irritability increased risk of… <ul><li>depression</li><li>PTSD</li><li>anxiety</li></ul>impaired focus impaired concentration impaired memory impaired learning abilities

	increased risk of dementia decreased reaction time
BEHAVIORAL	increased appetite decreased sexual arousal reduced motivation reduced job performance increased risk of auto accident increased impulsivity

Now that you know the risks of sleep deprivation, I encourage you to mark off all YOUR motivating factors for better sleep:
- Increased focus
- Reduced stress
- Improved memory
- Improved learning abilities
- Improved concentration
- Improved emotion regulation
- Decreased irritability
- Improved sexual desire
- Improved sexual functioning
- Increased lifespan
- Increased motivation
- Increased creativity
- Increased reaction times
- Improved coordination
- Improved job performance
- Decreased risk of heart disease
- Decreased risk of high blood pressure
- Decreased risk of certain cancers
- Decreased risk of type 2 diabetes
- Decreased risk of obesity
- Decreased risk of dementia

- Increased energy
- Improved skin elasticity
- Improved metabolism
- Decreased risk of depression
- Decreased risk of anxiety
- Reduced symptoms of posttraumatic stress disorder
- Decreased risk of dementia

IMAGINE: What would your ideal sleep schedule look like? What would your sleep quality look like? How would you feel waking up each day? How would you feel throughout the day?

What are your current "Sleep Busters?" Do you have any additional ones that weren't listed above?

What do your current sleep schedule and nighttime routine look like?

Okay, now we know WHY we want to get better rest, let's tackle the HOW:

"Sleep Boosters" – Healthy Sleep Habits

Use your bed and bedroom environment for sleep ONLY...with the exception of sexual and other intimate activities. That's right: your bed and bedroom environment are reserved for sleep and sex ONLY. If you are doing other things where you are supposed to be sleeping, you're going to confuse your brain and body!!! Here's what I mean by that. The more we do things in bed that are incompatible with slee–like reading, worrying, eating, watching TV, etc–the more we start associating the bed with these activities. That association will typically lead to some sleep difficulties.

Keep a comfortable sleeping environment and block out light and noise. We want to ensure that our bed and bedroom environment promotes restful sleep, so think dark, quiet, and cool. If there are noises or lights that you can't control (maybe the neighbors are throwing a raging party, or they have an obnoxious security light that shines right into your bedroom, or you have a snoring partner or pet), figure out what you can do to accommodate those disruptions! Try to reduce ambient light or noise by using earplugs, room-darkening curtains, or an eye mask.

Go to bed only when you're beginning to feel sleepy.
Suppose you routinely lie in bed tossing and turning at night, and it's taking you forever to get to sleep. After a while, your brain and body will associate tossing and turning with the place where you are supposed to be sleeping! If you are trying to force yourself to go to bed at a certain time–even if you are not tired– just to "get your eight hours," you're probably not doing yourself any favors.

If it takes you longer than 20 minutes to fall asleep, get out of bed and do something relaxing. Side note: that doesn't mean watching the clock to see how long you've been awake; going with a guesstimate is fine.

Get out of bed shortly after waking up. While it may be tempting to stay in bed and watch TV or scroll social media, remember that our goal is to rebuild the association between bed and sleep! Getting out of bed right after waking up will also help reduce your temptation to press the snooze button. If you are having trouble with this, I would again highly recommend reading Mel Robbins' book, *The 5 Second Rule.* In the book, she talks about how creating a mental countdown from five to one and immediately taking action has helped bust her habit of snoozing (seriously, Mel, I'm a HUGE fan!).

Take a hot bath or shower before bed. The warm water raises your core body temperature, so when your body begins to regulate back to a normal body temperature, you may begin feeling sleepy.

Create a relaxing nighttime routine. Turn off your tech devices at least thirty minutes before bed and start a wind-down routine that will help you decompress from your day. This helps to better prepare yourself for a restful night's sleep. This nightly routine will also help train your brain and body to recognize that it's almost time to go to sleep!

Don't watch the clock! This can actually reinforce your negative sleep thoughts. And, honestly, it doesn't do you any good to "calculate" how much sleep you can squeeze in—or how much you're losing out on if you don't fall asleep right at that moment!

Set a regular schedule for sleep and wake times. Our brains and bodies LOVE routine. A solid timetable for when you wake up and go to bed will help you get a more restful, restorative sleep! If you work night shift or any kind of abnormal shift work - I feel you and I know how tough that can be!

Get sunlight during the day! Exposure to natural daylight helps regulate our circadian rhythm, which plays a big role in our sleep schedule.

Catch a nap! A power nap can work wonders for you, but you must be strategic about taking one! It's best if your nap is in the early afternoon and only about twenty to thirty minutes (*and yes, I'd recommend setting an alarm for your nap time!*) That way, the nap won't interfere with your ability to fall asleep that night.

Avoid alcohol at least four hours before bed. Let me guess...you might be thinking, *But Melyssa, alcohol helps me fall asleep at night!* I have heard this more times than I can count...and I used to say it myself! That is until I started paying more attention to the effects of alcohol on my sleep quality. Basically, while alcohol may help you fall asleep at night, it actually impairs the quality of your sleep during the night! Consuming alcohol before bed also tends to lead to more feelings of drowsiness in the morning and the experience of "brain fog" during the day. Don't worry; we will talk more about alcohol in upcoming sections!

Avoid caffeine after noon. That's right, y'all: while we may love to start our day with a caffeinated kick in the booty, consuming caffeine after noon can impair our ability to fall asleep! This can happen because one serving of caffeine stays in your system for about six to eight hours, so consuming coffee after noon could keep you from falling asleep when you go to bed. Obviously, everyone has different sensitivities and tolerance levels to caffeine. Still, the general rule of thumb is to avoid caffeine (coffee, tea, energy drinks, and some chocolates) in the afternoon.

Get active during the day (especially in the morning!). Starting your day with movement is a great way to boost your energy! Also, daily activity, especially in the morning, helps you burn more energy throughout the day, which will help you feel sleepier at the end of the day.

Avoid heavy meals before bed, but don't go to bed hungry! If you need a pre-bedtime snack, try to enjoy a small serving of food that contains natural melatonin. Foods like strawberries, kiwis, almonds, and cherries can help boost melatonin to promote sleep.

Catch and Challenge Negative Sleep Thoughts! HUH?! I know you are probably thinking, "*Uhhh…Melyssa, how does the way I think affect my sleep?*" While I worked with clients on sleep health, I learned that negative sleep thoughts can be one of the most POWERFUL tools we have in our healthy living toolbox! Negative sleep thoughts are those nasty, unhelpful thoughts that say things like, *OMG, I'm NEVER going to get to sleep… I CANNOT go to sleep without my sleep med/supplement/etc… It's SO late already; I'm only going to get five hours of sleep if I go to bed right now, and I will be SO UNBEARABLE to be around!* None of those thoughts will help you fall back asleep and stay asleep. We need to learn how to CATCH then CHOOSE or CHANGE the negative thoughts we have about our sleep to stop them from interfering with our sleep! Let's dive in deeper and revisit some of our thought challenging skills from our Mindset Matters chapter…

COGNITIVE RESTRUCTURING

Unhelpful sleep thoughts can negatively impact our sleep health—it's true! I know, I was skeptical when I first heard about this too. To demonstrate how this works, let's look at an example:

I'm NEVER going to get to sleep!

How does that statement make you feel? Frustrated? Annoyed? Worried?? Having that thought only adds to our stress, which (as you now know) interferes with our sleep! Not to mention, we are likely to have these negative worry thoughts as we're lying in bed trying to get to sleep–also NOT helpful!

Like in other areas of our life, the unhelpful thought patterns, which affect our behaviors, can also show up if we have sleep difficulties. They may even worsen our sleep quality! Consequently, it's essential to understand some of the facts on sleep that can help you challenge those unhelpful sleep thoughts as they arise. So get ready to arm yourself with the knowledge to knock out those thoughts keeping you from your precious, quality sleep!

Know your sleep facts:

- People with sleep difficulties tend to underestimate the amount of sleep they get by almost an hour and overestimate how long it takes them to fall asleep at night too!

- Daytime sleepiness is normal throughout the day, especially 30-60 minutes after waking up and after lunch. However, people experiencing difficulty sleeping will view these typical pockets of daytime sleepiness with more negativity.

- Nighttime awakenings when you feel alert and awake are also normal. They will usually be followed by an onset of drowsiness shortly after. Nonetheless, people with sleep challenges will often view this normal experience more negatively and will experience more unhelpful sleep thoughts.

- While sleeping pills help people stay asleep, they do not help people fall asleep since it takes around 60 minutes for the medication to be absorbed by the body. People will often fall asleep faster after taking a sleeping pill, though, because they think it will help them to do so. (*See the kind of power our thoughts can have?*)

Let's work through some examples of unhelpful sleep thoughts together:

Unhelpful Thought	More Helpful Thought
"*I can't sleep without taking a sleeping pill!*"	"*Eventually, I WILL fall asleep, even without a sleeping pill. It just might take longer to fall asleep than I'd like.*"
"*It's going to take me FOREVER to fall asleep tonight!*"	"*It is still taking me longer than I'd like to fall asleep, but I am working on making changes to help me fall asleep faster!*"
"*I'll NEVER be able to go back to sleep now!*"	"*Feeling awake during a nighttime awakening is normal, but that doesn't mean I won't start feeling sleepy soon. I will probably fall asleep shortly!*"

What negative sleep thoughts have you had/do you have?

How would you change those to more helpful sleep thoughts?

ENGAGE

How important is it to you to make positive changes for your sleep health?

0 - 1 - 2 - 3 - 4 - 5 - 6 - 7 - 8 - 9 - 10
(*not at all*)   (*extremely*)

How confident do you feel in making positive changes for your sleep health?

0 - 1 - 2 - 3 - 4 - 5 - 6 - 7 - 8 - 9 - 10
(*not at all*)   (*extremely*)

What are some of your current habits that PULL YOU AWAY from healthier sleep?

What are some of your current habits that PUSH YOU TOWARD healthier sleep? What habits would you like to introduce that support healthy sleep?

What is *one* healthy sleep skill you could try today?

Chapter 6:

Stress Less

"If you are depressed you are living in the past...
If you are anxious you are living in the future...
If you are at peace you are living in the present."

–Lao Tzu

Choose the statement that best reflects your feelings about your current stress management strategies:

- I don't need to learn how to better manage my stress.
- I can't learn how to better manage my stress.
- I might learn how to better manage my stress.
- I will learn how to better manage my stress.
- I am learning how to better manage my stress.

In this section, Change Makers, you will learn how to stress less! Notice how I didn't say, "*How to be stress-FREE?!*" When you see those "*21 days to be stress-free!*" challenges, just know they are total bullshit. You will never truly be without any stress in your life (*nor would you WANT to be totally stress-free!*) Stress is actually something that helps keep us alive, so let's talk about stress, baby!

I'd love to start with my personal account of dealing with unmanaged chronic stress.

I was relatively healthy at 26-years-old, and I LOOOVED my job! I worked a lot of overtime, doing as much as possible because I wanted to excel in my career. Unfortunately, I ignored the signs my body was giving me, telling me I needed more rest. I was just in that "hustle" mentality, pushing myself to my limits. Ultimately, I ended up contracting Hand-Mouth-and-Foot disease—yep, those of you who are parents or teachers probably know this is common in preschool children, not adults. But here I was at 26, dealing with these weird itchy bumps on the palms of my hands, the soles of my feet, and in the back of my throat.

My doctor looked at me and said, "Have you been experiencing excessive stress lately?" And my reply was, "Nope, I'm not stressed! I love what I do. This is the happiest I've been in a really long time." However, as he explained, my body contracted this childhood disease because stress weakened my immune system. It also made me more susceptible to catching something my body would normally fight off.

I heard what he was saying, but I didn't really *listen*...

So after being out of work for almost two weeks waiting for the Hand-Mouth-and-Foot to clear up, I went right back to doing things the way I had before. Unfortunately, I didn't learn my lesson the first time, and my body decided to give me an even bigger wake-up call...I ended up with shingles—on the left side of my face! That's right, y'all—*my money maker was wrecked!!!*

The shingles virus had taken over my entire left facial nerve bringing along painful blisters on my mouth, nose, temple, and cheek. The blisters would crack and bleed whenever I tried to talk, smile, or eat. It was not only physically painful but also emotionally traumatic due to the insecurity I felt...I mean, it was like the Hunchback of Notre Dame level of shame. Or, perhaps, Phantom of the Opera, as I wished I had a half-mask to hide the hideous blemishes. I couldn't sleep because the entire left side of my face felt like it was on FIRE...I was in so much pain. I had to go out on short-term disability because I had no more vacation time at work (*NOT how I would have chosen to spend my well-deserved time off*).

I am sharing this story to encourage you not to let it get to that extreme before you listen to your body. When I share this story at speaking engagements, I usually have a few people tell me they've had similar experiences with illnesses that were stress induced. So, y'all, make sure you pay attention to the signals your body is trying to give you! As you listen, consider what changes or adjustments you might need to make to keep yourself healthy and happy.

Please know, however, that I'm not here to make stress the bad guy. Some stress is actually good stress! We can use stress to our advantage, so I don't want you to think that ALL stress is terrible for you. In fact, Dr. Kelly McGonigal does a fabulous job describing how our interpretation of stress can make it more or less harmful in her TED Talk and book, *The Upside of Stress*. As she points out, we NEED stress in our lives (*just not too much of it for too long…*) to help us stay safe. For example, if you were about to walk out into the road in front of a bus, your stress response would cause you to jump back out of the way and not become a road pancake. Since stress is something we have to live with, let's look at how to get GOOD at stress…

EMPOWER

First, we need to start with a reflection. I encourage you to take a few moments to answer the following questions…

What is stress?

What does stress feel like to you?

How does stress show up for you?

What is causing you stress?

While our bodies react the same way in stressful situations by activating our fight-or-flight response, the experience of stress can vary from person to person. Consequently, it's important to reflect on how stress feels to YOU. If you have a hard time identifying how stress feels for you, the list below may help you pay more attention to your stress symptoms. This is not an exhaustive list by any means; however, you can use it to mark off the symptoms of stress that YOU experience. Also, feel free to add your own.

PHYSICAL:
- Tension in shoulders
- Clenched jaw
- Tension in hands
- Diarrhea

- Racing heart
- Rapid breathing
- Increased sweating
- Gastrointestinal upset
- Increased sweat
- Fatigue
- Headache
- Decreased sex drive
- Bodily aches and pains
- Chest pain
- Other:
- Other:
- Other:

MENTAL/EMOTIONAL:
- Racing thoughts
- Increased irritability
- Feelings of overwhelm
- Impaired focus
- Impaired memory
- Difficulty concentrating
- Feelings of sadness
- Worry
- Emotion dysregulation (AKA: trouble managing emotions)
- Other:
- Other:
- Other:

BEHAVIORAL:
- Eating too much
- Not eating enough
- Sleeping too much

- Not sleeping enough
- Not exercising
- Restlessness
- Procrastination
- Alcohol, tobacco, and/or drug use
- Social withdrawal or isolation
- Impulse buying (AKA: "retail therapy")
- Other:
- Other:
- Other:

Please note any of your observations while working through this activity:

EDUCATE

Let's get to know our stress a bit better! There are many different types of stress, and understanding what each one is all about will help us in making the most of our stress!

EUSTRESS

Eustress is the GOOD kind of stress that helps to motivate you. For instance, this type of stress is experienced during physical activity, while preparing for an important event, or going on a first date.

DISTRESS

Distress is the BAD kind of stress and can be harmful or draining if not properly managed. This is the stress resulting from challenging life circumstances and unexpected difficulties such as health issues, the loss of a loved one, or financial strain.

ACUTE STRESS

Acute stress resolves when you are safe from a dangerous or stressful situation. Let me give you an example. You are driving on the highway, and some crazy cars are cutting you off. Then, you almost get sideswiped by this jackwagon weaving between the lanes going 30 over the speed limit! You slam on your brakes and yell profanities watching him continue to endanger the lives of other drivers on the road. What's happening in your body and mind at this moment? You just experienced a stressful event, and your body is probably amped up with your hands clenched on the wheel as you try to hold on for dear life. At the same time, you remain hypervigilant for the rest of your drive while you look for other yahoos that might pull a similarly stupid stunt.

When you finally make it to your destination, what happens? Your death grip loosens from the wheel, your shoulders drop out of your ears, you let out a sigh of relief, and maybe even your clenched buttcheeks start to relax. You've made it, and your body decides that you're safe. As that stress begins to resolve, the relaxation response kicks in to help you recover from the stress you've just experienced. That short, temporary burst is acute stress, and it helps to keep you safe in dangerous situations.

CHRONIC STRESS

Chronic stress, on the other hand, is long-term stress. An example of chronic stress could be caring for a sick family member...or the COVID-19 pandemic that we all just lived through. Chronic stress is the type that doesn't really resolve itself because of the ongoing nature of a situation. Instead, it causes your brain and body to be constantly on alert...hellooooo dysregulated nervous system! Since you're always looking for a threat or trying to protect yourself, your body's relaxation response continues to be suppressed as the stress response remains activated.

The biggest problem with chronic stress is that it can lead to many adverse health effects, just like my story demonstrates. Stress has a massive impact on our immune functioning, and after the COVID-19 pandemic, I think we can ALL agree that we want to keep our immune systems healthy and strong. Not only that, but unmanaged chronic stress can lead to other significant health conditions like heart disease, hypertension, and even certain types of cancers.

We need to recognize the toll that distress can have on our bodies and minds so that we may catch ourselves when we're beginning to experience elevated levels of stress. While it's essential to become more adept at recognizing increased stress, learning how to use stress management skills effectively is also crucial. And just like the stress response shows up differently for each of us, stress management skills will also work differently for each of us!

It's your job to become your own researcher with YOU as the test subject! So, try out different strategies to find what works best for you and your experiences of stress.

THE STRESS RESPONSE

During the stress response, also called the fight-or-flight response, our body kicks in all available resources to keep us safe, whether running from or fighting off danger. Obviously, that will cause a lot of physical strain as the physiological response to stress increases our heart rate, blood pressure, and breathing rate quickens. Our system is also flooded with a hormonal cocktail of biological "gasoline" that includes adrenaline, cortisol, norepinephrine, and other hormones pumped through our veins.

Let's take a moment to think of our body as a vehicle. When the stress response kicks in, our body "presses on the gas." It starts channeling our energy and resources to protect ourselves. But what happens if we keep that gas pedal floored and never give ourselves a chance to pump the brakes? Go ahead, take a guess! Imagine if you had an open stretch of freeway with no obstacles and ran your car with the pedal to the metal. What would happen over time…?

There could be many possible consequences here, like running out of gas or overheating the engine! After all, cars aren't built to function at that level of performance for an extended time, and neither is your body. So there will be times you need to ease off the gas pedal and slow down or even slam the breaks! And that's where the yin to stress's yang comes in…

THE RELAXATION RESPONSE

Ideally, our body activates the stress response when dealing with acute stress. After the stressful situation resolves, our relaxation response kicks in. This response works in opposition to the stress response, meaning that when the stress response gets activated, the relaxation response gets suppressed or deactivated, and vice versa. The relaxation response allows our brains and bodies to recover from the stress we've just experienced by reducing our heart rate and blood pressure, decreasing our respiration rate, and regulating our hormones back to baseline levels.

Chronic stress can become a problem if it frequently remains unresolved without allowing our relaxation response a chance to take over. Since the relaxation response counteracts the physiological activation of the stress response, its ineffectiveness means our bodies are left operating at a heightened state of arousal for longer periods. Just like in the metaphor of the body as a car, this can cause significant wear and tear if our body doesn't get a chance to repair the damages it experiences during that heightened stress.

It is also important to realize that how we all live nowadays also causes issues with our relaxation response. In our modern world, we respond to non-life-threatening situations the same way, and on the physical and physiological level, as we would to actual life-threatening scenarios. That means we may react to a missed work deadline the same way we would to being chased by a bear...even though we're *not going to die* because of a missed deadline. You can start to see the problem there, right? The way we think about certain situations is causing us more stress than we need to experience based on our perception of the situation.

THE EXPERIENCE OF STRESS

It's important to recognize that we could have varied stress responses to the same event based on our interpretation of its effect on our lives. Think about it this way: two people could be involved in the same car accident, and one could walk away a little shaken up and the other with a potential acute stress reaction that could eventually lead to posttraumatic stress disorder. Both people were involved in the same situation, but their *experience* of the circumstances was very different.

I'm not trying to say that we can simply make ALL of our stress disappear by changing our thoughts...but we CAN reduce our stress that way. We can change the amount of stress we experience by changing our interpretation of that stress. Check out the Stress Reappraisal section below for some examples!

STRESS AND BEHAVIOR CHANGE

Chances are that you might have learned how to deal with stress in ways that don't support your well-being. Unfortunately, we typically do not get to witness adults engaging in healthy coping strategies throughout our childhood. In addition, we have never been properly taught how to manage our stress in healthy ways. Usually, we engage in behaviors that help us avoid the discomfort of distress. For example, we might numb our problems away with alcohol or comfort foods. We could also avoid them by procrastinating, scrolling social media, or oversleeping. While these actions may provide temporary relief, do they ultimately support your well-being?

Just like we discussed in our section about dealing with our thoughts and emotions in new ways, we can also learn how to deal with our stress in ways that are aligned with our values and promote our health and well-being. It's essential to recognize how stress affects our choices and how we can become more aware of our stress response behavioral patterns. Let's take some time now to explore stress in your life, how you're currently managing it, and ways in which you can become more effective.

EMPOWER

What are some examples of eustress in your life?

What are some examples of distress in your life?

What is important to you about building effective stress management skills? How will this be helpful to you?

What ways do you currently cope with stress that do not support your health and well-being?

ENGAGE

Stress Reappraisal: Changing the way we think about stress can be an effective way of reducing the stress we experience. When we're stressed, we often revert to "worst-case scenario" thinking, which can cause us even **MORE** stress since we're stressing about what is stressing us out...AHHHH! Not the most helpful...so what can we do instead? The good news is that we have some amount of control over how much stress we experience, based on our interpretation of our experiences. Think about it this way–two people could be involved in the same car accident: one person walks away just slightly shaken up, the other person walks away and could develop post-traumatic stress disorder (PTSD). We can work to train ourselves to interpret our situations and sensations differently to help reduce the stress we experience.

View your stress experience differently	*"Oh no, I'm so stressed! This is terrible and harmful to my body!"*	*"My body is preparing me to handle this difficult situation and getting ready to support me through it!"*
Catch your unhelpful thoughts	*"This is the WORST thing that could be happening right now..."*	*"I notice I'm having the thought that this is the worst thing that could be happening right now."*
Reframe your stress into excitement	*"I'm so NERVOUS right now..."*	*"I'm so EXCITED right now!"*
ABCD method: **Activating event** **Beliefs** **Consequences** **Dispute**	*What is the event that triggered stress?* *What beliefs or thoughts come up?* *What are the consequences of those beliefs?* *How can you think about the event differently?*	*A: Missing a work deadline* *B: "I'm going to get fired!"* *C: Feelings of fear, distress, anxiety* *D: "I may get repercussions, but this is not a fireable offense."*

Practice Mindfulness

The Mindful Minute
Set a timer for 60 seconds while counting your deep breaths. Count each inhale/exhale as one breath. Take long, slow, deep breaths into the belly. After 60 seconds, remember the number of deep breaths you took so you can take a "mindful minute" wherever you are!

Body Scan
Find a comfortable position. Begin with a scan of your entire body, starting at the top of the head or the feet. Make observations about any sensations you feel without judgment as you move your attention from one area to the next. Try to relax each body part as you bring it to mind and focus your attention. Remember that your mind will wander, and that is okay. Patiently and compassionately refocus your attention back to the body, wherever you remember you last focused your attention. It's important to note that you may not feel any particular sensations in the body, and that's okay too! Just notice the absence of sensation as you go through the body scan meditation.

Progressive Muscle Relaxation
Create intentional tension in a muscle group as you take in a deep breath. You can try clenching your fists, raising your shoulders to your ears, flexing your feet, etc. Hold the tension and the breath for two to three seconds. Release the tension as you let out a long, full exhale. Focus your attention on the relaxation of the muscles as you let your breathing return to its natural rhythm. Repeat two to three times for each muscle group creating and releasing tension with each deep breath.

Visualization
Imagine yourself at a place where you feel peaceful and calm, such as the beach, mountains, or lake. This could be a real or an imagined location. Try to picture that place in as much detail as

possible, engaging each of your senses: what do you see/smell/hear/feel/taste? Allow yourself a few moments to immerse yourself into this place you've created in your imagination, inviting feelings of relaxation, peace, and calm.

Deep Breathing
Deep breathing helps us activate the relaxation response, down-regulating our nervous system.
Breathe into the belly for a full inhale, and release the breath through the mouth in a loud sigh.
Explore different variations of deep breathing, such as 4-7-8, box breathing, alternate nostril breathing, etc.

In the Resources section at the end of this book, I have a link to my website where you can find some of these practices as a special bonus!

Healthy Coping

Exercise
Whether it is an intense session of resistance training, a mindful walk outside, or an at-home dance party, moving your body can help shift your distress into eustress!

Journaling
Putting pen to paper can be a powerful way to process your feelings and thoughts about certain situations. Gratitude journaling can also work wonders for pivoting out of a doom-and-gloom spiral and shifting your focus to what's good in your life! We will discuss gratitude in greater detail in later chapters.

Social Support
Talking with friends, asking for help with tasks or projects, or just getting together for some enjoyable social outings can help you feel connected and supported, which helps to relieve stress.

Professional Support

If you find yourself overwhelmed and experience significant impairment in your daily functioning due to stress, reach out to a mental health professional. Remember, it is not a sign of weakness to ask for help. In fact, it is actually a sign of courage and strength. Going to therapy is a great way to learn new coping strategies. A professional can also help you address the causes of your stress through reflection, processing, and planning as they guide you through stressful times.

Healthy Snacks

While it is tempting to reach for comfort foods jam-packed with carbs and sugars, having healthy snacks can help you eat to beat stress! Giving your body nutritious foods can help reduce inflammation and increase feelings of well-being. Moreover, research is beginning to show us that a stomach can act like a second brain! Highly processed foods can trigger lethargy and depressive symptoms and increase susceptibility to stress. Meanwhile, unprocessed nutrient-dense foods can help buffer the effects of stress and support a gut microbiome that helps protect against feelings of depression, anxiety, and stress!

Breaking it DOWN

If you have an overwhelming project or task causing you stress, break it down into smaller, more manageable steps. This will help you focus on taking one step at a time and give you a little dopamine hit as you mark off each step along the way!

Worry Time

It might sound counterintuitive, but scheduling a specific time to worry as much as possible can keep worrying from taking over your entire day! Unless there is something time-sensitive and urgent, worry time allows you to notice your worry thoughts come up, but not focus on them until later. Try to have your "worry time" scheduled for 5-15 minutes in the early evening hours, so it's not too close to bedtime. During that time, you can journal or think about the worries that popped up throughout your day. You might be surprised that when you show up to your worry time, many of the worries you did have throughout the day don't show up again! You can also dedicate a specific spot in your life where you let your worrying take place. That way, you can "leave your worries" behind in that space!

What are some potential barriers you might encounter while practicing these skills?

What are some possible solutions to help you overcome those expected challenges?

How important is it to you to make positive changes in your stress management?

0 - 1 - 2 - 3 - 4 - 5 - 6 - 7 - 8 - 9 - 10
(*not at all*)   (*extremely*)

How confident do you feel in making positive changes for your stress management?

0 - 1 - 2 - 3 - 4 - 5 - 6 - 7 - 8 - 9 - 10
(*not at all*)   (*extremely*)

What are some of your current habits that *PULL YOU AWAY* from healthy stress management strategies?

What are some of your current habits that *PUSH YOU TOWARD* healthy stress management strategies? What habits would you like to introduce that support healthy stress management?

What is *one* stress management skill you can try today?

Chapter 7:

Choose Less Booze!

"Imagine what it would sound like if an alcohol commercial was required to list side effects like pharmaceutical drug commercials do...

WARNING: alcohol consumption may cause vomiting, diarrhea, weight gain, sleep loss, cringe-worthy embarrassment, blackouts, brain fog, heart disease, certain cancers, and–in some cases– death..."

–Melyssa Allen

Sensitive Topic Warning
- *Substance Misuse*
  - *Suicide*

Choose the statement below that best reflects your current feelings about your alcohol consumption:

- I don't need to make changes with my alcohol use.
- I can't make changes with my alcohol use.
- I might need to make changes with my alcohol use.
- I will make changes with my alcohol use.
- I am making changes with my alcohol use.

Take some time to write down what you know about the effects of alcohol consumption and our health:

PLEEEASE, I am begging you not to skip this chapter. Remember Change Makers, this book isn't about making us feel bad about our lifestyle habits! It's about helping us raise awareness of what is helping and what is hindering our health and well-being journey. Also, even if you don't drink alcohol, you might get some helpful information to share with the people you care about in your life.

Do you know what is so crazy to me?? I don't remember getting any kind of education on issues surrounding alcohol use (*besides the DARE: Drug Abuse Resistance Education program when I was a kiddo*) until my late twenties, when I enrolled in a Clinical Psychology PhD program and learned about substance use disorders. That class was an eye-opening experience for me as I learned what a standard-size drink was, the damage alcohol

159

caused to our brains and bodies, and what is classified as "high-risk" drinking behavior. What rocked my world even more, though, was recognizing how many of my family members–including myself–were engaging in what would be categorized as "high-risk" drinking. *Cuuuuue the instant denial*

The more I reflected on this new information, the more I wanted to resist it! Why were the healthcare organizations trying to demonize alcohol?! I saw alcohol as a great way to relax and unwind, and to feel more confident. For me, it was usually linked with a great time. After all, I was trying to have some fun and live my best college life in my twenties! Sure, there have been times when I went waaaaaay too hard and immediately regretted it, but that didn't mean I had a problem...did it?

Not necessarily... However, if alcohol is causing ANY kind of impairment in your life–with relationships, health, work, etc.– you may have a problem at hand. Many of us have an image of what a problem with alcohol "looks like." You may be picturing someone who needed to be hospitalized and had to have their stomach pumped. Or maybe you're thinking of someone who ended up with a DUI or blacked out. Yes, these situations can happen, but, truthfully, those are the extremes. Most of the time, problems can sneak up on you slowly and steadily, until you reach a breaking point and have a wake-the-fuck-up call. However that wake-up call looks for you, please make sure you pay attention to it.

Dad's Story

After learning about alcohol use, which we will get to shortly, I remember being worried about my dad. Back in 2012, his older brother, my Uncle Jerry, died by suicide. Unfortunately, it hadn't been Uncle Jerry's first attempt at taking his own life. He had had some serious struggles with anxiety and alcohol use over his lifetime. It was an extremely tragic event for our family, especially my dad. Uncle Jerry was a party animal. He was fun to be around and had an unmistakable laugh that was infectious! In hindsight, it hurts my heart to wonder how much of his personality was alcohol-induced because I have a hard time remembering a single time throughout my childhood when he wasn't drinking.

My dad also had his ups and downs with alcohol use throughout my childhood, but he never turned into an angry or violent drunk. Drinking was just how he decompressed after a long day of work as a delivery driver and how he bonded with his friends during his downtime. After experiencing a life-changing leg injury that resulted in chronic pain, my dad had to go on disability. I can imagine how he could have turned to alcohol to ease the pain and pass the time. I can also see how the habit of drinking to cope with that huge life change could have crept up on him.

Fast forward about 15 years to when I was in the PhD program and found the courage to have a conversation with him about my worries and the amount of alcohol he was consuming regularly. Despite feeling vulnerable, I shared that I wanted him to be around to walk me down the aisle and possibly play with some grandkiddos in the future! That was enough to plant the seeds. Eventually, he realized he wanted a change in his life too.

With how much and how long my dad had been consuming at the time, the safest route was taking him to an inpatient treatment center where he could have a medically-supervised detox. What is not common knowledge, is that alcohol withdrawal can be extremely dangerous for those who have been drinking heavily for prolonged periods of time. If a heavy drinker suddenly stops drinking, they can have a painful or even life-threatening state of withdrawal on their bodies. That is why I am so grateful and proud of my dad for taking that enormous step of courage to seek the help he needed.

And I know the entire story took only a few paragraphs to tell, but it took about eight months from our first conversation for my dad to ask me to get him help.. I'm so proud of him for taking that courageous step to start treatment. I know it wasn't easy for him. Honestly, it was scary as hell for both of us, but that entire experience brought us so much closer together and our relationship is better than I can ever remember.

After that experience, you'd think that I would get my shit together and limit my own drinking. Listen, y'all, I'm only human too. Can you guess what I did to escape, avoid, and numb my uncomfortable emotions and unhelpful thoughts? You got it! I tried to eat and drink my problems away... ironic, isn't it? I had just taken my dad to treatment for alcohol use and then used alcohol to cope with the situation. *YIKES*.

While my dad was in treatment, I was basically eating and drinking my feelings. I was going through a quarter-life crisis and questioning whether I made the right move joining a doctoral program. Especially after I was asked to bring a note from the treatment center when I dropped off my dad because I had to miss a midterm that day. I wish I were kidding, but I literally had to ask the treatment facility staff to print me a letter to "excuse" me from the midterm. Regardless, that was just one of the MANY things that led to my eventual transfer into the Clinical Psychology Master's degree program.

While I was enrolled in the Master's program, I also began working towards my board certification in lifestyle medicine. However, as I continued to study for the certification and further educate myself on the dangers of alcohol consumption. The knowledge I gained helped me take a good, hard look in the mirror when I had a health scare of my own.

My Own Wake-Up Call

At the end of 2019, I went in for my annual PAP smear exam, a procedure where cells are scraped from the cervical tissue to detect abnormalities. By this point in my life, I was used to having abnormal results, and it was almost something I had come to expect. But this time, the results showed that I had contracted HPV (human papillomavirus), even though I had had the HPV vaccination as a teenager. These cells became more aggressive and, eventually, precancerous.

I had to undergo a procedure to remove the precancerous tissues, but when I went back a few months later, I still had abnormalities. I felt scared and angry that the procedure hadn't "cured" me. At that point, I decided to try whatever I could to prevent this condition from getting any worse.

While I was dealing with my health issues, I was also learning more and more about lifestyle medicine. Because I was now desperate to try anything that would keep me from developing cervical cancer, I decided to eat more healthy, get back to regular physical activity, and significantly reduce my alcohol intake.

Do you know what happened after a few months of these lifestyle changes? *POOF*!!! "Miraculously," I had normal results at my check-up. This hadn't happened in close to 10 years!!! Of course, it now makes total sense to me: HPV is a virus, and viruses thrive off of inflammation. By participating in behaviors that reduced the inflammation in my body, I created an environment where the virus couldn't thrive! I must caution you, though. I'm not saying that all cervical cancers can be "cured" through behavioral change, but I can tell you from personal experience that healthy behaviors can reduce your risk and even prevent the onset of this type and some other cancers.

I'm going to bet that many of you can relate to some of these stories in some way. As you keep reading, it's important to continue extending compassion toward yourself. And if reading about these issues is stirring up some difficult things for you, please reach out to a mental health professional for support.

STAY WITH ME HERE...

This chapter might be bringing up some uncomfortable stuff for you, like it does for me. Still, please remember how important it is to reflect on the things we want to avoid most and to bring a sense of self-compassion and patience to this topic....

Do you remember when smoking used to be the "cool" thing to do? You know how, during earlier generations, smoking cigarettes and pipes was glamorized? But then, all these studies started coming out about the significant negative health impacts of smoking tobacco? And the deep pockets of the tobacco companies worked really hard to keep that research from being widely known because it would hurt their bottom line…And despite knowing that smoking was a public health crisis, the greedy politicians continued to promote smoking because they were getting funding from those tobacco companies? And then health organizations demanded that tobacco companies had to include warning labels on their products and fund public health education campaigns to raise awareness of the damage that smoking does to our brains and bodies?

Yeeeeah, well, unfortunately history is repeating itself with the current promotion of alcohol use. Eventually, more and more research emerged demonstrating the adverse health effects of tobacco use. It had even been suggested by the research that one in three cancer deaths would not occur if no one used tobacco products! In light of these findings, health organizations had to strongly advocate for including warning labels on packaging. There was also a slew of public health campaigns to raise awareness of the damaging effects of tobacco on the brain and body.

Alcohol ads usually show these sexy, beautiful people walking through a club in slow motion with a seductive look in their eyes on their way to the bar where they order up a glamorously luxurious drink. Or maybe you've seen the all-American ads showing friends tailgating at a football game and sharing a few beers? Or maybe you've seen clips of coworkers enjoying happy hour after a hard day of work? All of these instances demonstrate how normalized the consumption of alcohol as a means of socializing has become. And with this normalization, the rate of alcohol consumption—and alcohol-use disorders—have begun climbing.

Now, despite alcohol also being listed as a carcinogen, it is not experiencing a similar backlash. I don't see the alcoholic beverage companies advertising that their products could increase your risk of certain cancers by up to 40%. That's right, folks, I hate to burst the bubble—and, trust me, I was SOOOO resistant to really taking this information to heart—but alcohol is a class one carcinogen. This means it's classified at the same level as tobacco. Class one carcinogens are the substances and products that have the highest risk of increasing the occurrence of certain types of cancers. Alcohol is linked to increased rates of esophageal cancer, liver cancer, pancreatic cancer, stomach cancer, cervical and endometrial cancers, and (especially for women) breast cancer. Recent research has demonstrated an almost 8% increased risk of developing breast cancer with average alcohol consumption rates of LESS THAN one drink per day.

Basically, the more alcohol you consume, the higher your cancer risk. *YIKES!!!*

This information is not something that's widely publicized… why is that? I believe it all comes down to money. It's not in the best interest of alcohol manufacturers to advise people to start drinking less, because that means less money for them!

I know as I started learning more about alcohol's effect on our health and well-being, my eyes were opened to a whole wealth of information that I had no idea existed. Unfortunately, that's a pretty common occurrence, as we're told to responsibly enjoy ourselves without much mention of the negative side effects. Thankfully, many companies have started speaking out about the negative health effects that alcohol can have and have begun to offer non-alcoholic alternatives. I believe it's only a matter of time before we begin seeing the labels on alcohol include more than the "don't consume while pregnant" warnings like maybe a note about the increased risk of certain cancers.

It sucks, it really does, because this is one of those situations where the world is working against us to live our healthiest lives possible! And let's be clear, I'm not saying that you shouldn't EVER drink alcohol (*again, I am not about that deprivation lifestyle*). Don't get me wrong, I absolutely enjoy chilling at a craft brewery for date night and meeting up with friends! Sure, there are DEFINITELY some populations of people who should NOT consume alcohol, including those under the age of 21; those who might not have the best relationship with alcohol and can't control how much they consume; those who are pregnant; and those taking certain medications. If you don't belong to any of those populations and would like to drink occasionally, then by all means enjoy yourself!

And to be quite honest… I actually have to thank alcohol for giving me the courage to make the first move in my relationship with my boyfriend of almost six years! It was Cinco de Mayo, the margaritas were flowing, I treated the table to a round of tequila shots, and the rest is history! But as much as the liquid courage helped me find the confidence to take a giant leap of faith and risk rejection, I also could have done the same if I had just believed in myself. After all, I did not have to rely on those few drinks to dig up the confidence I already had inside! The moral of the story is that the "benefits" you think you are getting from your alcohol consumption are costing you waaaaay more in the long run…

I want to be clear that it's important for you to be mindful of how much you consume and to seriously consider making changes if you fall into the moderate to high risk categories. Many of us are blissfully unaware of our own drinking habits or the drinking habits of those we care for. And because alcohol is becoming a leading public health crisis, it's essential we start having this conversation right now.

EDUCATE

Alright, let's talk about why we should choose less booze. I'm not saying we have to quit altogether, although the recommendation for optimal health is that no amount of alcohol is "safe" to consume, but decreasing our intake of alcoholic beverages truly has many benefits. Various entities related to health, such as the Center for Disease Control, the American Heart Association, and the American Cancer Society, all recommend that if you're not drinking alcohol, you shouldn't start! But if you're already consuming alcohol, let's introduce some guidelines for lower risk drinking behaviors to help reduce adverse health effects.

BEER: If you are consuming beer , a 12-ounce, 5% alcohol by volume (ABV) beverage counts as a standard-size drink. If you've ever gone to a brewery, typical beers are served in pint glasses, which are 16 ounces. So there, you're already consuming more than one standard-size drink! Also, many of those craft beers are typically going to be over 5% ABV, so that's something to keep in mind too as you're tracking your consumption. Here's a tip: To slow down your consumption, alternate the beer with water. Alternating an alcoholic beverage with water, not only helps to slow down your consumption, but also provides your body with some assistance in metabolizing the alcohol that you do consume.

WINE: If you are consuming wine, a 5-ounce glass of around a 12% ABV wine is going to make up one standard-sized drink. Now, if you are anything like me, you are not paying attention to how much wine you are pouring yourself at the end of the day. At home, you don't typically measure out the wine or pay attention to the size of the glass, right? So, it's easy to say that you've only had ONE drink, even if the glass is huge. Therefore, unless you are at a restaurant that lists portion sizes, you will need to take steps to figure out exactly what a 5-ounce glass of wine looks like to understand how much you are drinking. Listen, I've used all of the excuses myself too, but the only person you are cheating is your future self, so don't skip this important step.

LIQUOR: If you are consuming a drink made with hard liquor, the standard-size drink measurement is 1.5 ounces of 40% ABV liquor. OK let's get real: If you are chummy with your bartenders, chances are you are going to get a pretty heavy-handed pour! Did you know that bartenders have a special tool they're supposed to use to measure out the shots? I don't know about your experiences, but the bartenders I see are often doing freehand pours. This means you can't really know how much alcohol you're getting in a single drink—you might even end up with two to three servings of a standard size-drink in a single glass!

OK, now that we've talked about what one standard-size drink looks like for the three different types of alcohol, let's talk about the amount of alcohol that is considered a "low-risk" daily and weekly drinking behavior. Here are the recommendations from the Dietary Guidelines for Americans:

WOMEN:
- No more than ONE standard-size drink on any given day.
- No more than SEVEN standard-size drinks within a week.

MEN:
- No more than TWO standard-size drinks on any given day.
- No more than FOURTEEN standard-size drinks within a week.

Men process and metabolize alcohol in their bodies a little bit differently, which is why their numbers are slightly higher than the recommendations for women.

OK, take a moment here to notice what's coming up for you. Does it seem like a ridiculous ask to cut your drinking by that much or does it feel doable? Take a moment to jot down some notes about your thoughts and feelings brought on by what you've just learned.

BINGE DRINKING:
You know the phrase, *"Work Hard, Play Hard"*? We are hard at work during the week, so we can party it up on the weekends, right?! Trust me, I am a HUGE fan of a bottomless mimosa brunch, for a good ole Sunday Funday! Unfortunately, that mentality of partying hard on the weekend is costing our society MILLIONS of dollars through healthcare costs, lost productivity at work, and accidental damages (CDC.gov). According to the CDC and recent research, binge drinking is the "the most common,

costly, and deadly pattern of excessive alcohol use in the United States."

To continue this conversation, we need to better understand what binge drinking looks like and what its negative health effects are on our brains and bodies. Here is a breakdown of what is categorized as binge drinking:

- FOUR drinks in a two-hour timeframe for women.
- FIVE drinks in a two-hour timeframe for men.

Keep in mind that these are **standard-size drinks.** Oftentimes, if you're out at a bar, you might be getting a single pour that is more than one standard-size drink. While you might be thinking you're only having three "drinks" at a craft brewery, if those drinks are pint-sized then you might actually be getting the equivalent of almost five standard-size drinks!

ALCOHOL AND OUR HEALTH:

- Did you know even low-risk drinking impacts our brain health? Studies have shown that heavy alcohol consumption is associated with brain atrophy, neuronal loss, and poorer white matter fiber integrity. That means our brain literally shrinks and begins losing some functioning. Recently, there have been even more studies examining how low-risk drinking can negatively affect our brain structure, health, and functioning.
- As I've previously mentioned, recent research is demonstrating strong links between alcohol consumption and rates of cancers. This risk is due to *acetaldehyde,* which damages your body's DNA and can cause your cells to grow in funky ways that could lead to the development of cancerous tumors.
- We all know liver health suffers with alcohol consumption, but other bodily organs and functions are also affected.

Your heart, pancreas, and circulatory and immune systems all take a hit when you drink alcohol.

- Alcohol is classified as a depressant, which means in addition to having physical effects on our brains and bodies, it also impacts our mental health. Alcohol use is connected to increased symptoms of depression, reduced cognitive functioning, and increased emotion dysregulation—like outbursts of anger.

EMPOWER

The first step in making change with your drinking habits is becoming aware of the exact amount of alcohol you are consuming without being judgmental. On my own journey, this has been one of the toughest reflections for me; it might be for many of you, too. Prior to learning about the negative effects of alcohol, I was just drinking it to enjoy myself without paying attention to how much of it I was consuming. For me, alcohol was an escape, a great way to decompress at the end of the day. But then, I was also using it to celebrate special occasions, too—so crack that bubbly and let's party, y'all! That means I was drinking to forget my problems AND drinking to celebrate the good times—so can you imagine how surprised I was when I actually began tracking how much I was drinking?!

And you know what? If you start becoming more mindful and aware of how much you consume, the amount you drink regularly might surprise you too! But remember to think about it this way: what are you sacrificing by choosing to drink regularly? You could be robbing yourself of a healthy relationship with the person you love or stealing away important years from your future self. You could be holding yourself back from a promotion at work because of the brain fog you have after a night of drinking. You could also be using the alcohol to numb your emotional or physical pain to the point that you are depriving your children of a present and attentive parent.

I would like you to take a moment to think now: is drinking alcohol worth sacrificing all of those other things in your life?

Important Note: Please make sure to consult a mental health provider if you are having a difficult time changing your drinking behaviors.

I want to take this opportunity to thank you for sticking with me through that chapter, especially if it felt uncomfortable for you to read about alcohol use and its risks.

Please take a moment to answer the following questions:

On average, how much alcohol are you consuming per week?

What are your motivating factors for consuming alcohol?

What are the costs (*both immediate and potential or long-term*) of your alcohol consumption?

Check off which of the motivating factors below are desired outcomes for changing your drinking habits:

- Reduced risk of cancers
    - Liver
    - Esophageal
    - Breast
    - Colorectal
    - Ovarian
    - Cervical
    - Prostate
    - Pancreatic
    - Kidney
- Reduced risk of heart disease
- Reduced risk of stroke
- Reduced risk of obesity
- Reduced risk of diabetes
- Reduced risk of Alzheimer's disease
- Reduced risk of dementia
- Reduced risk of high blood pressure
- Reduced risk of depression
- Reduced risk of accidental injury
- Reduced risk of high cholesterol
- Reduced signs of aging
- Improved sleep quality
- Improved immune system functioning
- Improved sexual desire
- Improved sexual performance
- Improved sleep health
- Improved memory
- Improved focus and concentration
- Improved productivity
- Improved energy levels
- Improved relationships
- Improved physical appearance
- Improved financial well-being through money saved
- Increased alertness

- Increased longevity
- Increased quality of life
- Increased savings on healthcare
- Increased positive emotions
- Weight loss

ENGAGE

By now, you might be wondering, "*OK Melyssa–you've told me to alternate drinking water between my alcoholic beverages… is that the ONLY thing I can do?!*"

I'm so glad you asked because there are sooooo many other, more creative ways to begin reducing your intake of alcohol! Here are a few strategies to consider:

- **Tracking your drinks:** Even monitoring how much alcohol you consume can reduce your intake! When we have to input the numbers, it forces us to recognize how much we are drinking. That simple action can lead us to drink less than we would if we weren't paying attention.
- **Working with a healthcare provider:** Ain't no shame in that asking-for-help game, y'all! Get a professional on your team–a professional who can help guide and support you with a personalized action plan for change! I can't tell you how many times I've had my therapist help me get unstuck with some of my self-sabotaging habits. (*Shoutout to you, Courtney!*)
- **Mindful drinking:** In the chapter on mindfulness, we learned to slow down and pay attention to the activity we were engaging in. The same guideline applies to drinking. For instance, nowadays, when I drink sparkling wine, I

don't just throw it back and chug like I used to for getting a quick buzz. Instead, I take a moment to turn my full attention to the experience. I watch the bubbles travel up the sides of the glass, notice the tiny firework show happening at the surface as the bubbles pop, enjoy the aroma, take that first sip, and then follow it from my mouth into my throat, down my esophagus, and into my stomach! Being mindful when drinking not only allows me to savor the experience but also to decrease my alcohol intake.

- **Track your symptoms:** It's going to be much harder to change your habit of drinking if you're not noticing the immediate effects on your well-being. So try tracking your mood, bloating, cravings, energy levels, etc., to see how alcohol affects your body and mind.
- **Choose non-alcoholic alternatives:** There are numerous companies releasing non-alcoholic beverages to help support the movement. Give them a try! You might be surprised that the taste makes it seem like you're drinking a regular glass of wine or pint of beer!
- **Try a sober streak:** Experiment with how long you can go without having an alcoholic beverage while tracking how you feel!
- **Urge surfing:** Typically, when we're trying to change habits, we will have urges that pop up after being exposed to a Cue. Before engaging in the Behavior part of the Habit Loop, notice what's happening for you in that moment. Instead of acting upon the urge, "surf it" and see if you can let it pass.
- **Explore joining a sober/sober-ish community:** If being around others is your Cue to start drinking, see if you can join any communities that gather over activities other than alcohol!

What are some strategies you can use to reduce your consumption of alcoholic beverages?

What are some obstacles you anticipate when it comes to changing your drinking habits?

In what ways would your life improve if you cut out alcohol completely or moderated your drinking to low-risk guidelines?

What habits could you introduce that support no to low risk drinking?

What is *one* skill you could try today to lessen your alcohol intake?

Now that we've talked about choosing less booze, our next conversation will center around...

Chapter 8:

Let's Move!

"If exercise could be packed in a pill, it would be the single most widely prescribed and beneficial medicine in the nation."

–Dr. Robert N. Butler

Choose the statement that best reflects your feelings about your current level of physical activity:

- I don't need to move my body regularly.
- I can't move my body regularly.
- I might move my body regularly.
- I will move my body regularly.
- I am moving my body regularly.

When it comes to using lifestyle behaviors as medicine for our minds and bodies, movement is one of the fastest ways to give ourselves a boost! I say movement here because many of you might view the terms "exercise" or "workout" in a negative light, and it might make you want to close this book–but wait, please don't! I'm talking about just moving our bodies, and doing so in whichever way you enjoy moving!

For some of you, that might look like a really high intensity interval training (HIIT) class that ends in sweat dripping into your eyes, your heart pounding in your chest, and the accomplished feeling of *"YES, I DIDN'T DIE!"* For others, it might be a mindful yoga class that allows you to focus on your breathing and enjoy some gentle movements to stay connected to the here and now.

But maybe you're thinking to yourself, *"OK Melyssa,I KNOW I should be exercising more, but I just find it feels like TORTURE!"* Well Change Maker, my favorite follow-up question to this is: What is it about physical activity that makes you feel miserable?

For me, as I'm currently at my heaviest weight, I find that the majority of my self-imposed misery comes from my own mind. The thoughts I'm hurling at myself while moving and trying to do something good for my health can be suuuuper negative. Do you know what else I've found? It can be extremely uncomfortable trying to find workout clothes that you feel confident in when you're a bigger size.

Let me tell you, I have been so tempted to start a sports bra brand that has cute patterns, sexy back designs, and provides the support that larger-chested women like me need, so we don't give ourselves a black eye from our boobs slingshotting towards our faces while we're trying to do jumping jacks! OK, maybe that is a slight exaggeration, but let me tell you what isn't: your boobs trying to suffocate you while in a Downward Dog pose during a yoga class! I mean honestly, y'all, it can be a serious struggle!

OK, rant over—let's get back to what makes exercise so miserable.

EMPOWER

If you believe that exercise is not enjoyable, take a moment to list your thoughts that contribute to that feeling or make you avoid exercising altogether:

What came up for you during that reflection? Did you notice a flurry of unhelpful thoughts that keep you from doing something that supports your mental, physical, and emotional well-being? What about some of those cognitive distortion categories we discussed in the Mindset Matters chapter—did you recognize any of those in there?

Chances are you did. This is where CATCH then CHOOSE or CHANGE comes in! We often have excuses such as lack of time, motivation, discipline, willpower, etc., that keep us from taking action committed toward our values! Take some time now to figure out which skills you are going to use to take the power away from those thoughts or to change them into more helpful thoughts:

ORIGINAL THOUGHT	CHOOSE or CHANGE

How did it feel to work through those thoughts? Use these newly transformed thoughts as your way to overcome those pesky excuses as they show up!

EDUCATE

As we move forward, I'd like to encourage you to shift your mindset away from "forcing" yourself to move in order to improve something with your physical appearance and toward using movement to promote your health, and then work on finding fun ways to do that!

Think about the kinds of activities you enjoyed as a kid.
Did you have a trampoline in your backyard and spend HOURS jumping the day away in your childhood? If so, what if you gave a trampoline class a try?!
How about roller skating? Maybe you spent hours at the roller rink trying to catch the eye of that cute boy or girl you were crushing on, waiting to impress them with your cool skate moves? What if you were to grab yourself a pair of skates and hit the rink again?!

We forget to allow ourselves an attitude of play in our adulthood. This can often rob us of the joy we could experience if we gave ourselves permission to act a little goofy now and then! Why did we start taking life so seriously as we got older? Sure, we have a lot more #adulting to do and more responsibilities to take care of that we didn't need to worry about as kids, but shouldn't that mean we're allowed to have even MORE fun?!

Finding the joy in movement again was one of the reasons I was so grateful to fall into group fitness classes. There is nothing like matching the energy of a room full of people all putting in their best effort, the bass from the music pumping so loud it feels like a second heartbeat, and the group all cheering each other on throughout the class. For me, there is NOTHING like leading a group fitness class that is beat-based; I like to say that any movement that is "musically-motivated" is my fitness love language! If you want to read more about the group movement experience, Dr. Kelly McGonigal shares some incredible stories and research findings in her book, *The Joy of Movement*, about the metaphorical magic created when humans are all moving synchronously with each other and the feeling of connectedness it creates among us.

Now, let's look at our mindset around movement again. We really need to focus on promoting our health by moving our bodies. If we solely rely on changes in our physical appearance for our motivation, we are going to be sorely disappointed! It can take weeks, months, or even YEARS to see the physical changes we desire, so we need to shift our focus to what's working for us in the short term—and that's going to be how we FEEL versus how we LOOK.

Sure, appearance goals can motivate us to a certain extent, but focusing on fighting to change our bodies can also make us lose steam REALLY fast. When it comes to changing these behaviors for the long haul, shifting our focus to the immediate benefits we receive from moving our bodies will make us A LOT more likely to follow through with building consistency. Remember the Habit Loop? Emphasizing that instant REWARD we get from choosing to move, will help reinforce the Cue(s) and Behavior!

So let's shift our focus from fighting so hard to change our bodies to learning how to work WITH our bodies instead. Shifting this focus will help us create a fitness routine for LIFE and not just one for that special occasion that we want to look hot and sexy for, like a wedding, summer trip, high school reunion, etc.

EMPOWER

What are the ways your body craves to move?

What is your body capable of?

How can you honor your body's current boundaries while working to push past your own limits?

EDUCATE

Let me start this next section by saying ANY amount of movement is better than none. Can't find the time for a 30-minute workout? That's OK, just find time to move for five to ten minutes! As you continue reading, please don't feel overwhelmed or discouraged by the numbers that follow. Remember, our focus is on progress over perfection! We just want to be able to start moving and keep moving to promote our health and well-being.

Check out this list of the benefits of regular physical activity and check off which ones could motivate you to start and stay active:

- Reduced risk of:
  - heart disease
  - stroke
  - colon cancer
  - breast cancer
  - esophageal cancer
  - prostate cancer
  - pancreatic cancer
  - obesity
  - arteriosclerosis
  - kidney cancer
  - diabetes
  - endometrial cancer
  - sleep apnea
- Reduced body fat percentage
- Reduced triglycerides
- Reduced risk of high blood pressure
- Improved blood flow
- Decreased risk of clogged blood vessels
- Reduced risk of high blood sugar
- Improved sleep
- Improved stress resiliency
- Reduced pain
- Lowered resting heart rate
- Improved immune system functioning
- Reduced risk of erectile dysfunction
- Improved sexual desire
- Decreased chance of weight gain

- Decreased risk of fatal heart attack
- Reduced risk for hip fracture
- Reduced risk of dementia
- Improved finances through decreased healthcare costs
- Improved performance and productivity
- Improved relationships
- Increased longevity
- Increased quality of life
- Improved confidence levels
- Improved self-esteem
- Improved body image and relationship with your body
- Increased energy
- Increased positive emotions
- Reduced emotional tension
- Reduced symptoms of anger
- Reduced symptoms of depression
- Reduced symptoms of anxiety
- Increased cardiovascular endurance
- Increased muscular strength
- Increased flexibility
- Setting a good example for your family

Isn't it amazing how beneficial movement can be? I bet you'd like to experience at least some of those benefits, right?

Well, then, let's dig into the nitty gritty details for movement!

AEROBIC ACTIVITY

The national recommendations for physical activity from the American College of Sports Medicine (ACSM) Exercise is Medicine® Initiative suggests the following:

- We should aim for 150 to 300 minutes per week of moderate-intensity activity

OR

- 75 to 150 minutes per week of vigorous-intensity activity

Initially, that sounds like A LOT, doesn't it?! Let's break this down a bit more to better understand what this means. During moderate-intensity activity, your heart should be pumping quite a bit, and you're probably going to get a little sweaty, but you could still have a conversation with someone! It wouldn't be a smooth conversation because you would be slightly out of breath, but you could still communicate efficiently! You wouldn't be able to hold a conversation if you were working out at a level of vigorous-intensity activity, though! During vigorous-intensity activity, your heart should be pumping heavily, and you should be huffing and puffing because you'd be so out of breath!

Now let's break down those numbers, so they are less intimidating! For the moderate-intensity activity guidelines, if you move five days a week for 30 minutes per day, that's going to get you to that 150 minutes per week benchmark! You could also spread that out even more throughout your week–it all adds up! ACSM actually published a great study looking at sprinkling exercise "snacks," or short bursts of activity, sprinkled in throughout a busy day!

I would like to take a moment now to pause and ask you to think about what you consider physical activity. What does physical activity look like for you? Chances are, you might actually be moving your body in a way that counts toward the recommended weekly time and not even realize it. So let's say you take your dog on a walk–your body is moving, and your heart rate is pumping a little bit more…and you're on your way to reaching your physical activity goal!

Structured physical activity is really beneficial, but ANY movement counts, and it all adds up over time. If you can find ways to incorporate movement throughout your day, even if it's a 10-minute walk while you're on your lunch break, you will easily reach your weekly goal. So if, in the past, you were able to carve out 45- to 60-minutes a day to fit in your workout routine, but no longer have the time, just go for that 10-minute walk. Those 10-minutes are better than none, after all. So focus on bringing back that progress-over-perfection mentality, and enjoy some exercise "snacks" as you build a sustainable fitness habit.

RESISTANCE TRAINING

You should participate in resistance or strength training at least twice a week, making sure you are not working the same muscle groups on consecutive days. Strength training can help maintain bone density and burn fat. Surprisingly, not many people know that building muscle also burns fat!

Strength training is based on the idea that you need to fight against a resistance. The resistance can come from your own body weight, gravity pulling on the weights in your hands, or tension from the resistance bands you're trying to stretch. When our muscles engage and contract against that resistance, we form teeny tiny little tears in our muscles. That's why we don't want to stack the same muscle group training days back-to-back–working the same muscles on consecutive days doesn't allow our body to heal and repair those microtears. Ultimately, not allowing your body the time to repair can contribute to injury. So please be mindful when scheduling resistance training sessions and remember to incorporate plenty of flexibility training.

FLEXIBILITY AND BALANCE TRAINING

Another important component of a well-rounded fitness routine is muscle recovery through flexibility and balance training. Our muscles spend so much time contracting during strength-based exercises, that it's important to give them a chance to stretch back out and release that tension! Flexibility allows our bodies to lengthen out our muscles that tend to stay contracted and can help relieve pain. Flexibility training also helps us age more gracefully because it can support our mobility, making it easier to preserve full functionality and range of motion. Improving our balance can also better prepare us for the aging process as it plays a key role in fall prevention.

This part of the book could be an entire chapter in and of itself, so if you are curious to learn more, make sure to check out the resources at the end of this chapter.

All the knowledge in the world won't help us to move, though, if we don't change our relationship with movement and continue avoiding it. I know I've used nearly every excuse in the book to avoid my workouts, *"I'm too tired… I don't have time… My workout clothes are dirty… I just ate… I haven't eaten yet!"* It's time for us to bust through those thoughts by using our strategies for getting untangled and by engaging in a process called Behavioral Activation.

That's right, y'all, Nike had it right with their slogan to just freaking DO IT and so did Mel Robbins with her 5-Second Rule. Both of these strategies focus on taking ACTION, *regardless of what you are thinking and how you are feeling at the moment,* and can help people push past their thoughts and feelings that keep them stuck.

It doesn't have to be much movement either–focus on a "bite-sized" amount to help you get started! In fact, The American College of Sports Medicine (ACSM) has done research on "exercise snacks," which are quick bouts of vigorous movement for less than one minute–findings have shown even those small "snacks" can improve cardiovascular fitness levels!

In fact, there have been times when I've told myself, *"I'll just walk for five minutes..."* and before I know it, those five minutes turn into ten, ten into twenty, and twenty into thirty! Perhaps quoting Newton's law would be appropriate here: An object at rest, stays at rest unless acted upon by an outside force. And you don't want to continue being an object at rest!

EMPOWER

What can you use as that "outside force" to help yourself bust out of a rut and make those first few moves to create positive momentum?

What does your current level of activity look like?

How could you move more throughout your day?

How could you transform movement into something you look forward to and find enjoyment in?

ENGAGE

How important is it to you to make positive changes so that you could get regular physical activity?

$$0 - 1 - 2 - 3 - 4 - 5 - 6 - 7 - 8 - 9 - 10$$
(*not at all*)   (*extremely*)

How confident do you feel in making positive changes so that you could get regular physical activity?

$$0 - 1 - 2 - 3 - 4 - 5 - 6 - 7 - 8 - 9 - 10$$
(*not at all*)   (*extremely*)

What are some of your current thoughts and behaviors that PULL YOU AWAY from regular physical activity?

What are some of your current thoughts and behaviors that PUSH YOU TOWARD regular physical activity? What habits would you like to introduce that support regular physical activity?

What is *one* strategy that you could try today that could help you enjoy regular physical activity?

We now know movement can act as medicine for our minds and bodies. Hopefully, you've started considering new ways of both seeing and doing activity in your own life!

And now... I've saved the "best" for last: the topic that throws everyone's panties in a bunch! That's right folks, we've reached the part of this healthy living book where we discuss–*drum roll please...*

Chapter 9:

Good Mood Food

Let food be thy medicine
and medicine be thy food.

–Hippocrates

Choose the statement that best reflects your current feelings about your nutrition:

- I don't need to make changes with my nutrition
- I can't make changes with my nutrition.
- I might need to make changes with my nutrition.
- I will make changes with my nutrition.
- I am making changes with my nutrition.

POP QUIZ! (*Just kidding, you're not getting graded on this*).
True or False: Dietary risk factors are the second leading cause of mortality for lifestyle-related chronic diseases.
(*Keep reading for the answer!*)

We've now reached the most confusing section of this book–WTF should I eat?! Remember Change Makers, I am not a registered dietitian, so I will not tell you what you can and cannot eat because your diet can depend on SOOOOO many different factors! Instead, what I will be sharing is an overview of the research conducted on the link between food and mood, the recommendations for healthful eating, and some thoughts on the patterns around our eating behavior.

Before we move on, though, let's take a moment to recognize some of our unhelpful thoughts around nutrition. Please, take some time to reflect on what you tell yourself when it comes to healthy eating.

I would also like to address some of the common phrases used to help "motivate" people to change their eating habits such as *"Nothing tastes as good as skinny feels! You are what you eat! A moment on the lips, a lifetime on the hips!"*

UGGGGGH... These phrases literally make me want to throat punch whoever is saying this shit out loud anymore. I will admit, though, when I was going through my disordered eating and exercise addiction phase, I shared quotes like this all the time because I wanted soooo badly to be "sexy" and "beautiful." After all, I saw these phrases in all the magazines that advertised what to eat to get skinny and I fell for them. But truly, thanks to our toxic and unrealistic societal beauty standards, aren't we all being conditioned to believe that skinny equals sexy AND healthy?

The truth is that there is still a stigma around people with bigger bodies being classified as "unhealthy." In reality, body size does not necessarily correlate with how healthy you eat. You could be eating shit all day every day and be skinny, or you could be eating according to the recommended nutritional guidelines for healthy eating and be bigger-bodied. But which version of you do you think would be viewed as the "healthier" one based on your physical appearance?

Fortunately, there are now movements dedicated to raising awareness around the fact that "healthy" doesn't look a certain way or is a certain size. I've been a fan of the Healthy at Every Size® (HAES®) principles for the last few years. I only wish I would have known about the concept when I was in my phase of peak physical fitness performance. The principles would have helped me realize that I could be "in shape" even if I didn't have bulging biceps or six-packs abs and didn't "look like" a gym rat. So I'm going to ask you a favor: Can we pleeeease ditch the toxic dieting phrases?

You are SO much more than what you eat.

Another important point to consider is the proliferation of toxic "health" and "fitness" industries. These industries have saturated the world with edited photos of muscular bodybuilders and airbrushed skinny models to paint a picture of "perfect" bodies. In addition, many of their fitness plans preach unrealistic messages like, *"Just don't eat (insert popular food item) and you'll drop weight in no time!"* or *"Follow this (insert fad diet) and you'll lose weight for life!"*

First, we are unique human beings, and there is no one-size-fits-all approach to nutrition. Second, chances are, you will gain the weight back as soon as you start reintroducing those forbidden foods. Finally, our bodies and brains **need** macronutrients like healthy fats and carbs, which are often the target of those "lose weight quick" campaigns.

Can we PLEASE stop demonizing the food we eat?

Can we PLEASE stop viewing certain foods as "bad" or "junk"?!

OK, sure, there are foods that our bodies need, and foods that we want. Now we realize that A LOT of different factors contribute to our relationship with food and eating. Still, ultimately, it comes down to our mindset around our food, how we eat, and what we eat that can help us work toward making more positive changes. It is time to work on healing our relationship with food and shifting the way we think about it, so that we can, once again, see it as medicine, fuel, and a source of enjoyment linked to our well-being! In addition, because we frequently try to "out-eat" a poor exercise routine, or "out-exercise" poor nutrition habits, we also need to look at the link between our mindset regarding both nutrition and activity.

Food is fuel for our bodies, and to fuel our bodies, we need to have the proper fuel to perform and function optimally! If we revisit the metaphor of your body as a car, we can say that we can't give a premium car low-grade fuel–that's going to cause ALL kinds of problems!!! And let me just STOP that negative self-talk before you even go there: *But what if my body IS an old beater and rejects the premium fuel?!* Do you honestly think I'd ask you to make a super drastic and overwhelming overhaul to your nutrition overnight...??

HELL NO, Y'ALL!

I would hope you know me well enough by now to know that is **definitely not** how I roll when it comes to changing behaviors and habits. OK, with that being said, we're going to start with some simpler, smaller changes to give ourselves a confidence boost and then build up from there! Before you know it, that "old beater" of a body of yours is going to be enjoying mid-range fuel and then, eventually, premium fuel ALL DAY long!

But let's face some harsh truths for a quick second. In today's world, the odds are working against us. Not to sound like a conspiracy theorist, but there are people out there who are paid to figure out how to make foods more addictive! It's true, y'all, snack companies LITERALLY hire psychologists and neurobiologists to figure out how to make their foods more addicting (just like social media, right?!). SO CRAZY... but that's why we need to become aware of the various influences affecting our choices and behaviors.

Oftentimes, we use food to comfort us, which can lead to emotional and/or stress eating. Not only that but we can actually develop real food addictions because there are so many additives in our foods. These additives give us this nice little hit of dopamine whenever we eat them. In addition, the added artificial flavors are hyper-palatable, which means they're **bursting** with flavor–usually sugary, salty, and/or savory. The flavors tingle our taste buds and make us want MORE! So basically, we are working against the odds when it comes to eating more healthfully (*but hang in there... there IS good news, I promise!*).

Take it from me, I have sooooo much unlearning to do still when it comes to healthy eating behavior. Middle school "me" used to devour three microwavable single-serving mac and cheese meals in one sitting. Present day "me" can still eat her way to the bottom of an entire family-sized bag of potato chips in a single day! And yet, here I am writing this book for you about healthy living... pretty wild, right? Because even though there are times when my cravings and mindless munching get the best of me, I have reached a point where the majority of the time I am fueling myself with foods that nourish my mind and body. I've learned how to make room

Remember to approach the following sections with open-mindedness. Try to notice any unhelpful thoughts that come up for you and get yourself untangled from them. Please remember, show yourself acceptance and compassion as we move through this information, because you are here to learn and grow!

Are you ready?! OK, y'all, let's start digging into the nitty gritty details.

EDUCATE

Recommended Guidelines: *The Nutrition "North Star"*

The Whole Food Plant-Based (WFPB) Lifestyle:
DON'T FREAK OUT, Y'ALL! I am in no way telling you to become a vegan or vegetarian here. Trust me, as a recovering barbecue addict from the heart of Texas, I have not completely given up my red meats, and I'm not asking you to do that either.

PHEW!

OK, now that we've got that out of the way, the whole food plant-based eating pattern is like the North Star for nutrition. The WFPB lifestyle promotes optimal health by swapping out some of the animal products and processed foods we eat for plant-based foods that look like they just came off the tree, out of the ground, or off the bush they grew on.

And while real plant-based foods are the most healthful, there is a massive uptick in food products promoted as "plant-based" while, in reality, they are heavily processed and only masquerading as healthy items. So as you reach for plant-based burgers or bacon, or other "healthy" but processed items, be mindful of the ingredients list. If the food has more than five things listed on its ingredient list, you may want to avoid it! Unfortunately *(sticking with the healthy choices aren't always the easy choices theme here...)*, there are A LOT of processed foods out there that are cheap, easy to make, and easily accessible. So we are going to work on making our whole, plant-based foods easier to make and more accessible.

But what IS the whole food, plant-based (WFPB) lifestyle? According to the American College of Lifestyle Medicine (ACLM), it's defined as *"an eating pattern that emphasizes a variety of nutrient-dense, minimally processed vegetables, fruits, whole grains, beans and legumes, and nuts and seeds."*

This may sound drastic at first, but when you look at the current MyPlate nutrition graphic from the USDA, it's not much different from a WFPB plate:

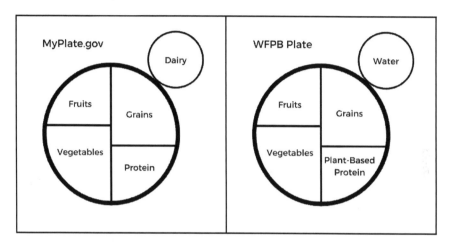

See? Whole food, plant-based eating really isn't so scary!

But I know what you might be thinking—*I know fruits and veggies are good for me, but it's expensive to eat healthy!* This is another common objection to healthy eating—how much it costs. We tend to think that eating healthier foods means spending more money, so let's tackle this unhelpful thought by reframing how we view spending money on healthier foods.

You may actually find that eating healthfully is cheaper over time because, as we consume more health-promoting foods, we can greatly reduce our risk of chronic diseases! So while it may be more of an investment initially, over the long term, healthy food could potentially save you a lot more money on things like medications, surgeries, or the management of disabilities. So if you find yourself saying, *"Eating healthy is too expensive,"* please remember to revisit your values and connect with how healthful eating fits into your Life Map. Ultimately, an investment in your health and wellness in the here and now will add up significantly over time—not only in money saved on health expenses, but also with your increased quality of life.

Some helpful strategies to save money while eating healthy:

- **Use frozen produce**: In some cases, frozen produce might have more nutrients than its fresh counterpart. Frozen produce is harvested at peak freshness and flash-frozen on the spot, preserving valuable nutrients, so keep in mind the seasonality of foods when shopping.
- **Consider canned/jarred options**: As long as the food is not drowning in oils or sugars inside the can or jar, these items can be great cost savers!
- **Buy in bulk**: With proper planning, buying in bulk can be a great way to save money on food!
- **Cook in batches:** Making meals ahead of time that you can freeze for later helps to reduce food waste. You can batch-cook your veggies, grains, beans, etc., so you can just mix and match your meals throughout the week instead of having to cook each night!
- **Reduce eating out**: Between the cost of the meal itself and tipping your waitstaff, eating out can add up quickly! Instead of eating out regularly, find ways to pack your lunches or prep dinners ahead of time. Save eating out at restaurants and fast-food spots for a special occasion!

I mentioned it briefly in the Choose Less Booze chapter, but red and processed meats are actually classified as carcinogens–known substances that increase the risk of cancer. TheCancer.gov website states:

"In 2015, based on data from 800 studies, IARC classified processed meat as a human carcinogen(Group 1), meaning that there is enough evidence to conclude that it can cause cancer in humans. The evidence for red meat was less definitive, so IARC classified it as a probable carcinogen (Group 2A)."

I don't know about you, but this was news to me when I was obtaining my board certification in lifestyle medicine. This news was also a HUGE wake-up call for me, especially since I was raised in a state where barbeque was treated like its own food group. I had never known that red and processed meats were grouped in with substances like tobacco and alcohol in terms of the damage they can cause to our health!

We started this chapter with a pop quiz. Here's the answer: **Diet is actually the #1 modifiable risk factor for lifestyle-related chronic diseases.** Many of the lifestyle medicine legends, like Dr. Dean Ornish and Dr. Caldwell Esselstyn, to name a few, have found that food can be "prescribed" to patients and used as "medicine" to prevent, treat, and even reverse conditions like heart disease, type 2 diabetes, hypertension, and more! How cool is that?! Sometimes I think we forget the power of nature in our lives, and eating whole, plant-based foods is one of the ways we can support our bodies and minds to function at their best.

FOOD FEEDS MOOD

There is considerable evidence that supports how the foods we consume impact our bodies. In fact, emerging research is now showing that foods can also affect our brains through the gut-brain connection! The research examining how the gut microbiome can act as a "second brain" is gaining some significant traction as I'm writing this chapter, but there is still a lot more that we need to learn. But we certainly can't deny the fact that eating certain foods can make us feel a certain way.

Sometimes, I indulge (*aaaaand maybe overindulge*) in a good Sunday Funday brunch jam-packed with processed meats like bacon and sausage alongside a bed of hashbrowns topped with an egg covered in cheese and end up feeling sleepy. Shoot, just writing that out makes me want to take a nap! Obviously, eating calorie-dense and nutrient-poor foods tend to contribute to feeling lethargic and bloated with a side of brain fog.

On the other hand, when I eat a power salad, I feel freaking UNSTOPPABLE–like my body is a temple, and I am the epitome of health and well-being. I also notice my energy is more sustained, and I don't feel groggy and foggy during the day.

Here's why this information matters…

The Standard American Diet (*SAD–yes, even the acronym admits that the Western dietary lifestyle makes you feel sad as your body processes all those calorie-rich, nutrient-poor foods*) has greatly contributed to many of the lifestyle-related chronic diseases we face today. As a result, the vast majority of health organizations, such as the American Cancer Society, the Center for Disease Control, and the American Heart Association, have released statements based on dietary guidelines that support health with the common theme being: **Eat More PLANTS!**

When we are constantly consuming highly processed, calorie rich, nutrient poor foods, it contributes to increased rates of inflammation in the body. Inflammation is a key player in lifestyle-related chronic diseases as we've touched on a bit already. It has also been suggested that inflammation is also linked with increased rates of mental health conditions, like depression and anxiety. While it may not result in the onset of these conditions, it can exacerbate some of the symptomatology you may be experiencing. Inflammation can create an environment that promotes the growth of harmful gut bacteria.

There is some fascinating research lately looking at the link between fruit and vegetable intake and ratings of positive emotions like happiness! In one study of 80,000 individuals from Great Britain conducted by Blanchflower et al. (2013), after controlling for additional factors known to influence emotional well-being, the researchers found an association between consuming at least seven to eight servings of fruits and vegetables per day and feelings of happiness... which lasted into the following day! Follow up studies have continuously supported findings that people who consume fiber-filled, plant-based foods show greater emotional well-being ratings!

As much as I wish *JUST* eating more plants was enough to help us flip the happy switch, that's unfortunately not how life works. But following a plant-based lifestyle CAN help give you a greater sense of empowerment. Plus, modifying your eating habits can help support your mental and emotional well-being!

EMPOWER

Check off all of the factors that would motivate you to make positive changes to your nutrition:
- Reduced risk of cancers
- Reduced risk of heart disease
- Reduced risk of stroke
- Reduced risk of obesity
- Reduced risk of diabetes
- Reduced risk of Alzheimer's disease
- Reduced risk of dementia
- Reduced risk of high blood pressure
- Reduced risk of depression
- Reduced risk of high cholesterol
- Reduced signs of aging
- Reduce risk of sleep apnea
- Reduced body fat
- Reduced insulin resistance
- Reduced inflammation
- Improved immune system functioning
- Improved blood sugar levels
- Improved sexual desire
- Improved sexual performance
- Improved sleep health
- Improved stress management
- Improved memory
- Improved focus and concentration
- Improved productivity
- Improved energy levels
- Improved relationships

- Improved physical appearance
- Improved financial well-being through money saved
- Increased alertness
- Increased longevity
- Increased quality of life
- Increased savings on healthcare
- Increased positive emotions

What else not on this list could motivate you to make positive changes to your nutrition?

Brainstorm some ways you could start adding more plant-based foods into your life:

ENGAGE

REDESIGN YOUR PLATE

Just think: When you go out to eat at a restaurant, what does your meal typically look like?? Does your order have an animal-based protein as the "main star" of the dish, followed by a "supporting actor" of heavy or fried carbs, and maybe the "guest appearance" of a vegetable that has been lathered up in some kind of oil? Honestly, I feel like our typical "American" meal has turned into a big ole burger with a heaping pile of fries and a beer on the side! I would also like to point out that portion sizes at restaurants and fast-food chains are usually OUTRAGEOUSLY oversized compared to what our delicate human bodies need!

So how about this—can we "recast" our plates to make our whole, plant-based foods the star of the show, with special guest appearances by meat and dairy? Again, you don't have to drastically redesign your plate overnight, but here are some strategies that could be helpful:

- Put your fruits/veggies/beans on the plate first so they take up the most space.
- Choose one meal out of your day to change up your plate portions.
- Find plant-based alternatives.
- Mix in some foods that you know you like with some new things you want to try.
- Try to have a variety of colors on your plate, so you can "eat the rainbow" throughout the day! Different colors of foods provide different vitamins and minerals, so while you might not have the entire rainbow on your plate at each

meal, try to eat a variety of different colors throughout the day.

What other strategies could you try to redesign your plate?

PHYSICAL VERSUS EMOTIONAL HUNGER

It's time you get to know your hunger signals! There are two types of hunger: physical and emotional. As their names imply, physical hunger is when your body is telling you, *"Hey! I need some sustenance over here!"* to meet physical needs. Emotional hunger, on the other hand, is *"Hey...I'm feeling bored, wanna eat some chips?"* Emotional hunger shows up when we're either avoiding uncomfortable emotions–like stress and boredom–or seeking out a pleasurable experience! Getting to know your hunger "hints" will help you determine whether you are physically hungry or craving something emotionally. Please don't ignore your physical hunger cues though–if you're hungry, grab a snack or a bite to eat!

CATCHING YOUR IMPAIRED EATING CUES

I don't know about you, but when I have a few drinks in me or if I'm watching TV, I turn into a bottomless pit! Not only that, but when I'm at a party, I gravitate toward the snack bar and end up continuously grazing on everything in sight! I like to refer to these as "impaired eating" choices, because they're made from a place of distraction and indulgence.

Once we learn to recognize the cues that lead to the behavior of "impaired eating," or mindless munching, we can take different actions to avoid those behaviors. Personally, I now try to put a few items on my plate and intentionally place myself away from the snack bar, so I don't keep grabbing and grazing! I'm also working on not eating in front of the TV and only eating at the dinner table, so I can retrain my brain and body to recognize that meals happen at the dining room table and ONLY the dining room table! If I do decide to snack in front of the TV, like while watching a movie, I do my best to portion out my snacks in advance. With portion control, I can ensure I'm only eating my way to the bottom of one serving of potato chips versus devouring the entire bag!

Another time impaired eating shows up for me is when I am RAVENOUSLY hungry, and I want to eat anything and everything in sight! If that happens to you too, make sure that you are checking in with yourself throughout the day to catch your hunger before it becomes uncontrolled. You could try using a hunger scale to monitor your level of hunger. I like using a scale of one (ravenous) to five (pleasantly full) to figure out how hungry I am. Over time, I've learned that if I'm below a three, I will most likely overeat to make up for the time I spent being hungry!

Reflect on the cues that cause you to make "impaired eating" choices.

Identify some strategies you could use to make alternative choices when you encounter those cues in the future.

80/20 RULE
Our brains can be so weird sometimes, especially when we tell ourselves, *"I can't have that..."* The more we fight the temptation,

the more we CRAVE it! So when you're learning to make healthier choices, try the approach of cutting back on certain foods instead of completely cutting them out of your life. This technique is called the 80/20 Rule. The framework suggests that 80% of the time, we should eat foods that nourish our bodies, and the other 20%, we can eat foods that feed our souls! Another way of thinking about this is that you're giving yourself permission to "treat yourself" around 20% of the time.

Please notice, I used the term "treat" and not "cheat." I prefer the former because it carries a more positive connotation. When we think about "cheating," we could experience feelings of guilt or shame, and that's the opposite of what we want to feel! So next time you allow yourself a little indulgence, think about it as a "treat" meal or a "treat" day! If you incorporate a bit of flexibility into your approach, you could find eating healthy to be a lot more enjoyable AND sustainable than you first thought.

80% FULL RULE (FROM BLUE ZONES)
Since we've been raised with the "clean your plate" mentality for generations, we're probably going to eat our poor bellies to capacity and feel miserably full. Let's take a page from the Blue Zones healthy lifestyle framework and work toward eating until we're only 80% full. And let's learn to avoid that after Thanksgiving Day dinner feeling when our bellies feel like they're going to BURST because we've reached capacity!!!

MINDFUL EATING
This strategy comes down to paying attention to what you are eating, while you are eating it. When eating mindfully, try to notice things you normally wouldn't be paying attention to. You could focus on the weight of the fork in your hand, the path of the food as it moves from the plate toward your mouth, the smell of your meal as it reaches your lips, your mouth watering in anticipation of

a bite, or the sensation of chewing. Mindful eating can help you slow down and make more careful nutritional choices.

Here are some helpful prompts for eating mindfully:
- Think about the journey this food took from its place of origin to your plate.
- What can you see? What can you smell? How many different flavors can you taste?
- How slowly (*while being safe!*) can you eat this food?
- What happens inside your body while you eat? How does your body feel? What sensations or movements do you experience?

KEEPING HEALTHY FOODS ACCESSIBLE
You know the phrase, "out of sight, out of mind?" We can use that idea to keep our "treat" foods out of sight while moving our "need" foods front and center! If you keep your healthy foods at eye level, you will be more inclined to reach for them when your hunger hits. And if you prepare healthier foods and snacks ahead of time, you will be more likely to reach for them as opposed to those highly-processed, fast food snacks when you are in need of something quick to eat!

FOCUSING ON ADDING MORE POSITIVES
To follow the theme of this entire book, focus on adding more health-promoting habits to your cooking repertoire.
Could you sneak some spinach into a yummy peanut butter and banana smoothie? *You betcha!*
Could you make a delicious bolognese with lentils mixed into the sauce? *You sure can!*
And could you add some mushrooms to your ground beef burgers? *100%!*

Remember, the more we focus on what we're trying to remove from our lives, the stronger our cravings will be. Shifting our focus from what we should avoid to what we could add to support our health can have a compound effect over time and lead to better nutritional choices!

Now that we've discussed five of the six pillars of lifestyle medicine, it's time to explore how social support can help us on our lifestyle-change journey to...

CHAPTER 10:

Stopping Slips from Becoming Slides

I didn't fail; I found out 2,000 ways how not to make a light bulb.

–Benjamin Franklin

Let me go ahead and burst your bubble, y'all–you *are* going to slip up at some point. I know I've already mentioned this a few times before, but what I haven't mentioned yet is that you can keep those temporary slips from becoming permanent slides. Now Change Makers, what I mean by that is just because you slip up doesn't mean you have to throw away all your hard earned-progress. It's funny how we become our own worst enemies when we try our hardest, especially when we're trying to create positive habits. For some reason, we tend to get in our own way!

So in our last discussion on lifestyle medicine pillars, I'd like to share how positive social connections can stop our slips from turning into slides. After all, strong social support can keep us more encouraged, more confident, and more accountable. And all those things are important when we're working toward becoming our best selves!

We want to surround ourselves with positive people who cheer us on and encourage us even during our toughest times instead of those who try to hit us when we're already down. Sometimes those positive people are hard to find, but chances are–if you're reading this book–there's someone else out there on the same page, with the same book in their hands, longing to find that sense of community to help push and motivate them toward reaching their goals and creating a life they love! You will be able to find those readers in our Change Maker Community, listed in the Resources section at the end of this book.

EDUCATE

Let's go ahead and discuss some of the benefits of social connections and why they're important. When we are around other people who uplift us and make us laugh and smile, we experience a release of a feel-good hormonal cocktail into our brains and bodies! All those happy hormones and neurotransmitters lead to some pretty significant health benefits. However, on the flip side of that, if you find yourself in a position without those strong social supports, you may experience some health complications.

In the list below, check off the benefits you would like to receive from positive social connections:

- Increased oxytocin
- Activated reward system in the brain
- Increased accountability and social support
- Lower blood pressure
- Decreased rates of chronic disease
- Increased rates of survivorship in cancer patients
- Increased resiliency
- Reduced feelings of loneliness and isolation
- Decreased inflammation
- Improved cardiovascular health

During the COVID-19 pandemic, loneliness and isolation took an especially significant toll on mental and emotional well-being. As humans, we're not meant to be alone! We are social beings and crave interaction with others, which is why so many people ended up adopting pets during the lockdown.

And while animals are amazing to have around, we are meant to be connected with other humans, first and foremost. If you look back at our evolutionary history, earliest humans formed tribes to keep safe. Within those tribes, people took on different roles that played to their strengths. Ultimately, that is where our urge and desire to *belong* stems from—it is what helped our ancestors survive!

So if you're thinking about sustainable, successful lifestyle changes, you're going to need some support. Whether it's professional one-on-one help from a coach or therapist, or support from a community with similar lifestyle-change goals, or help from your friends and family, it's important you have a team standing behind you!

I think it's safe to say that many of us have people in our lives who try to hold us back from becoming our best selves. You need to allow yourself to rise above their attempts to sabotage your progress on your journey to change. Obviously, that's going to be a lot easier said than done, but learning to set effective boundaries, communicating how you feel, and making appropriate changes in your relationships will help protect you and safeguard your progress.

It's also important to identify those charismatic individuals who energize and uplift you whenever you are around them! Perhaps

YOU are a charismatic individual in someone else's life? These energizing interactions will help support you in creating that upward spiral of positive momentum.

Like I've mentioned earlier, group fitness classes are one of my favorite places to be because the energy in the room is unmatched. Everyone moving together and working toward busting their own barriers to change in each class is something that I find so magical! There is so much power in the energy of the group experience, and if that's something you enjoy, you can use that energy as motivation to keep showing up, even when you don't feel like it–ESPECIALLY when you don't feel like it!

As research has shown us over and over again, support communities are key to helping us reach our goals. I don't know about you, but that is 100% true for me! On my own, I can let myself off with every excuse in the book and not feel a twinge of guilt... but the moment I have someone relying on me to show up? I will do whatever it takes to not leave them hanging!

Why can't I do that for myself though? I don't know... I'm still learning how to build motivation from within. But you know what? That's OK, because I have people willing to support me and keep me accountable for showing up–for them AND for myself!

That community support is a tool I am so grateful to have. It's also a tool that helps me immensely when it comes to reaching my goals–like writing this damn book...! Shout out to Dr. Moira Hanna for setting up coworking calls in the morning to help get my ass out of bed and seriously hunker down when I was only 90 days out from publishing! And you know who else I have to thank? (*Besides my editor, whom I have TOTALLY put through the wringer when it came to finishing this friggin book! Seriously Mar, you are the most AMAZINGLY talented and patient human ever!)*

I have YOU to thank–you, who is holding a copy of this book in your hands. Turns out, I do not enjoy the writing process whatsoever. I still don't consider myself a writer even after this whole grueling process! Honestly, I wanted to quit SOOOO many times but I kept telling myself that if this book could change even one person's life–it would have been worth it.

So thank you, dear Change Maker, for being there for me and helping to hold me accountable for following through with this book-writing process… even though you didn't know it at the time!

EMPOWER

I want you to take a moment now to think about these questions:

Who supports you and is your biggest cheerleader for your lifestyle-change journey?

How can you ask that person to be on your team? And what are some ways you can ask them to help support you along the way?

Take a moment now to think about some of the best relationships that you've had in your lifetime:
What did those people do for you? How did they show up for you?

What qualities did you respect most about them?

Now, I'd like you to think back to moments when someone was in need, and you were there for them:
In what ways have you encouraged others in your life? How did you show up to support them?

What are some of your barriers to building positive social connections?

- Technology
- Lack of self-confidence
- Lack of interpersonal skills
- Reluctance to interact with others
- Poor communication skills
- Fear of change
- History of unpleasant interactions
- Lack of time
- Social anxiety

What strategies could you use to overcome those barriers to positive social connection?

ENGAGE

Cultivating more positive social connections and interactions through enhancing your current relationships and building new ones can help you feel like you are part of something *bigger* than yourself while you're on your wellness journey.

Here are a few strategies that can help improve your social well-being:

Joining a community with a shared interest: Whether it's a spiritual community, a class that teaches a new skill, or a fandom, people who share similar interests can be helpful in fostering feelings of belonging. Interacting with people who are interested in the same things as you, will most likely lead to meaningful conversations and stronger bonds!

Volunteering for an organization or a meaningful cause: Chances are people volunteering for a particular cause will either have shared life experiences, similar values, or shared interests. In addition to cultivating relationships, volunteering has a slew of other benefits. For instance, when you're volunteering, you are likely to get a mood boost from participating since you're supporting a cause that is meaningful to you. You are most likely also going to experience a sense of accomplishment after the event! Because of all the positive outcomes, volunteering, along with Acts of Kindness, falls under the umbrella of positive psychology and fits in nicely with the PERMA model.

Creating micro-moments of positive connection: Sometimes, it just feels good to offer a smile or a little wave to a stranger. Those little moments of connection can convey the message of, *"Hey, I hope you're doing well today!"* and brighten someone's day. Really, any sign of kindness towards another human can be beneficial (the world needs more kindness anyways!). But even connections with pets, nature,or whatever you identify as a higher power can help you feel more engaged with and connected to those around you. The takeaway from this tip: be a good human!

Writing a relationship gratitude letter: We often forget to share with those we care about most what we appreciate most about them! Writing a letter of gratitude, or even a brief positive note, to someone you love can have a significant positive impact on your relationship! Here are some additional prompts you can use:

- Thank you for being my…
- I appreciate you because...
- I think you are special because…
- You make me laugh when…
- I have fun with you when…
- A favorite memory with you is…
- You are important to me because…
- When I think about you, I feel…

Giving someone you love a hug: I know people who consider physical touch as their love language–like this girl right here!--had a difficult time during the pandemic isolation. And while hugging others is best, if you find that you are in need of a hug and nobody is around, you can actually give yourself a hug. Research has suggested you will still receive some of those same benefits!

Remember to be your own best friend during your lifestyle-change journey, too, and invest in your relationship with yourself. Staying connected to your authentic self will prevent burn-out, especially if you're an introvert. I know I've gone through periods where I felt like I lost myself and then had a hard time finding myself again.

If you ever feel like you've lost a part of yourself, too, take some time to reconnect with who you are, what your values are, what's important to you, and what you enjoy most out of life. I hope that this helps you find ways to not only stay connected to yourself, but also to enhance your current and future relationships.

And all of this begins to come together and accumulate into creating...

Chapter 11:
Your ACTION Plan

If you fail to plan, you are planning to fail.

–Benjamin Franklin

Y'all—WE MADE IT!

We reached the final chapter of this book!

And while this is the final chapter of the book, Change Makers, this isn't the final chapter of your story. You are only beginning this lifelong process of learning, growing, and creating the life you desire, the life you deserve. Remember that you deserve health and happiness. No matter what you've been told in the past, no matter what you've told yourself over time, please remember:

You are worthy.

You are worthy of your dream life.

You are worthy of living a life in which you thrive.

You deserve to live a life in which you flourish.

This final chapter of the book brings everything together into one glorious action plan for lasting lifestyle changes. A plan that is created for you, by you. A plan that is based on everything that you have learned and the activities you've completed along the way. This is your go-to guide for setting your foundation of positive health habits that will add up over time to your total lifestyle transformation!

And yes, you're going to encounter obstacles.

And yes, you're going to face challenges.

And yes, there are going to be times that you fall flat on your face.

But none of those things matter unless you let them. What actually matters is each time you overcome that obstacle, you crush that challenge, and you pick yourself up again, dust yourself off, and get back to work! You get to create your secret recipe for success, and sometimes you will nail it on the first attempt and, other times, you will totally botch it!

Picking up where you left off each time you lose your way is going to be crucial throughout this journey. As the old saying goes, if you have one flat tire, are you going to slash the other three? No way–you fix the tire that's broken! And it's perfectly fine if you need to change the plan or change your goal along the way, just don't give up completely. Allow yourself to be less rigid around your goals and plans.Give yourself permission to be more flexible with your approach and try new things, troubleshoot through your challenges, and continue to explore what works best for you.

Revisiting your WHY

What is important to you about making lifestyle changes?

What is important to you about your previous answer?

What is important to you about your answer above?

What is important to you about your answer above?

What is important to you about your answer above?

Write a personal mission statement for your healthy lifestyle journey using your answers from the prompts above to serve as a reminder for why you are embarking on this journey:

Throughout these next prompts, you will begin building your ACTION plan for change! As you get down to the goal-setting and habit-change sections, I would reeeeeally encourage you to focus on one–and only one–aspect of your health and well-being. Pick something that you feel both motivated and confident to change. This way, you can put your full time and attention into changing that one habit to help you reach your goal! Instead of half-assing a bunch of things trying to change multiple behaviors at once, try putting your WHOLE ASS into changing that *one thing!*

I know it can be tempting to focus on more than one area of your health and well-being at a time. However, as we've seen throughout this book, all of these aspects of our health and well-being are interconnected: Getting physical activity helps us get better sleep, better sleep helps us manage stress more effectively, less stress leads to healthier food choices, healthier food choices lead to increased feelings of well-being, and on and on and on! That's why starting with ONE focused behavior–your foundation habit–can be enough to start a ripple effect through other areas of your life. Focusing on one habit will also prevent your time and energy from getting split between multiple behaviors simultaneously. Also, starting with one behavior allows you to establish a solid foundation you can later use to build other positive health habits..

Now, if you do want to try and tackle more than one habit or goal at a time, make sure to set that foundation habit first. Once that habit is firmly in place, you can add in "extra credit" habits. Here's the catch–your foundation habit is your priority–your #1 focus–and when you achieve it, you need to celebrate it! If you decide to set "extra credit" for yourself, think of it as bonus points only. So regardless of whether you accomplish your additional habits or not, if you've completed your foundation habit, you get to celebrate! However, if you miss your foundation habit, it's time to troubleshoot:

- **REFLECT:** What happened to keep you from following through with your foundation habit? Was there anything that prevented you from forming this habit?
- **REFOCUS:** Why are you working to change this habit in the first place? What is your purpose behind making this change?
- **REDIRECT:** What needs to change in your action plan to better help you follow through with this habit? Do you need additional resources? A stronger cue? A better reward to incentivize yourself?

This method can also be applied when setting your weekly and monthly goals. Sometimes you need to change the goal, and sometimes you need to change the plan–it's up to you to determine which route you need to take!

Your ACTION Plan:

What do you feel most *motivated* to change in your life?

What do you feel most *confident* to change in your life?

Let's revisit your Life Map from the beginning of this book...

VALUES
What are your values? What are the qualities you want to embody? How do you want to "BE" in the world?

GOALS
What are some of the goals that will help you achieve milestones aligned with your values?

Think about exactly one year from today–what would you hope to accomplish by then?

What could you accomplish in the next three months to help you move closer toward that goal?

Set a process goal for yourself using **either** the SMART goal framework or the FITT lifestyle prescription:

SMART Goal Framework:

S–Specific: What specific behavior/action are you focusing on?	
M–Measurable: How will you measure it?	
A–Achievable: How will you set yourself up for success?	
R–Realistic: How confident are you that you can achieve this goal?	
T–Time-Bound: When will you work on this goal, and for how long?	

Write out your full SMART goal:

FITT Lifestyle Prescription:

F–Frequency: How often will you perform this behavior?	
I–Intensity: How long will you perform this behavior?	
T–Time: When will you perform this behavior?	
T–Type: What is the behavior?	

Write out your full lifestyle prescription:

HABITS

What are the habits needed to support you in reaching your value-aligned goals?

What habit can you focus on to be the foundation for your change journey?

Once you decide on your foundation habit, complete the Habit Loop below and fill in your answers:

- **CUE(S):**

- **BEHAVIOR:**

- **REWARD(S):**

How will you track your foundation habit?

What unhelpful thoughts can you expect to face along the way?

What are some ways you can CHOOSE to get untangled from those thoughts or CHANGE the unhelpful thoughts into more helpful ones?

What uncomfortable emotions can you expect to face along the way?

How can you accept and make room for those emotions without letting them steer you off course?

What are some phrases you can use to remind yourself of your WHY, practice compassion and kindness towards yourself during a setback, and help you get back on track?

What tools will you use to support your lifestyle-change journey?

If you find yourself struggling with the goal you set above, how can you make it slightly easier?

How will you celebrate your successes along the way?

**Download your free action plan guide and additional handouts at healthylivingdoesnthavetosuck.com/bonus

CONCLUSION

Well, Change Makers—I can't tell you how much I appreciate you joining me on this journey toward better health and happiness! While I wish I could have offered every single behavior-change strategy that exists, I did my best to offer the ones I've seen work well for others and for myself. There are so many different ways to accomplish behavior changes, and I hope you are able to explore and discover the ways that work best for you. My wish for you is that this book helps you learn to accept your starting point and shows you how to trust yourself while you experiment with the various skills and strategies we discussed. I also hope that it shows you how to stay true to yourself and approach yourself with support, patience, and kindness as you work toward making lifestyle changes.

I'd like to wrap up by emphasizing some key takeaways from our time together....

- Use your action plan to focus on the next 12 weeks and give yourself enough time to experience how these smaller action steps add up to create larger lifestyle transformations.

- Stay connected to your mission statement and revisit your WHY to help you continue choosing value-based actions—even when you don't feel motivated or inspired.

- Remember to celebrate your wins—no matter how small—each and every time you make a choice and take an action that pushes you closer toward your desired future self.

- Focus on your accomplishments—this will create that upward spiral of positive momentum on your lifestyle-change journey!

- **The numbers on the scale do not define your worth** or accurately reflect your effort as you strive to adopt positive health habits—please find other ways of tracking your progress in addition to your long-term goal for weight loss.

- Take advantage of your strengths and reflect on what has worked well in the past to help you build new positive lifestyle changes.

- Feel all the feels! I know that you may be experiencing a whole mash-up of emotions right now: motivation, inspiration, fear, confusion, etc. Remember, those emotions all have their place, and it's our job to just let them come along for the ride as we work to build positive habits that support our health and well-being! Practice your self-compassion, self-kindness, and acceptance skills to help make this happen!

- You are NOT your thoughts! Use and continue to explore strategies for getting untangled from those unhelpful thoughts. Instead of letting your thoughts drive your behaviors, use your behaviors to help change your thoughts! Phrases like, *"Just Do It"* or *"5-4-3-2-1-Go!"* can remind you to take action before your mind talks you out of it with all those excuses!

- Continue cultivating that inner cheerleader to help support and encourage yourself through the setbacks and slip-ups! Even when that inner drill sergeant pops up again and again.

- Use the activities rooted in positive psychology to help give yourself a boost when you need it and also help you get unstuck from a rut.

- Find ways to bring lifestyle medicine into your everyday life and use these reminders to help:
  - *Sleep Well.*
  - *Stress Less.*
  - *Choose Less Booze.*
  - *Move More.*
  - *Eat More Plants.*
  - *Create Positive Connections.*

- Find your tribe and teammates to cheer you on along the way! If you need some extra support, please join our Change Maker Community listed in the Resources!

- Don't forget to consult with your healthcare providers too. They can provide you with valuable information and also connect you with resources that could help you reach your lifestyle-change goals.

- Ask yourself, "What is the *smallest* step I could take today to support my health and happiness?" when you find yourself struggling with motivation. Maybe it's drinking enough water for the day, taking your vitamins, eating a banana—some days you may only be able to commit to the smallest action. That tiny step forward is better than falling into a giant backslide!

I can't wait to hear about your incredible successes along the way and I hope you will share them with me! I am hopeful that this book will become a resource you can return to and I hope you will visit the book website for handouts of the exercises and activities. If you found this book helpful, the biggest compliment I could ever receive is for you to share my book with those in your life who you feel would also benefit from it! I appreciate you allowing me to share in this part of your journey with you, and I look forward to keeping in touch online!

Until next time Change Maker…
Take care, stay healthy, and be well,

Melyssa Allen, MA, CHWC, DipACLM

ACKNOWLEDGEMENTS

First and foremost–I would like to thank my dog, Buddy, and my kitten, Jackie. Without continuous pet therapy from these two blessed creatures, this book would have never happened!

Next, I want to give the BIGGEST shoutout to Matt for constantly supporting me through this process via shoulder massages, glasses of wine, and delicious dinners. I owe him back so much of my time that has been dedicated to completing this book after many anight spent in front of my computer screens. Matt, I can't tell you how much I appreciate you for your patience with me throughout writing this book! I honestly would have shriveled up from starvation if you hadn't taken care of me the way you did! I LOVE YOU SO MUCH!!!

Mom & Dad (*AKA: Susan & Bobby*), thank you for always believing in me and my crazy dreams and supporting me through the tough stuff! I've never had to question how much you both have believed in me over the years, and for that I am forever grateful. You are the most amazing parents in the world and I love you both soooo very much!

The rest of my family–Papa & Bama, my cousins, my friendship family members–thank you all so much for your patience and understanding with this big dream of mine! I know I have had to sacrifice precious time that we all could have spent together, and to know that you love me–even though I was absent–means the world to me.

To my closest ladies–Rose Marrone, Elyse (Paske) Benham, Kendall Menard, Nicole Uibel, Jess Ruiz, Kim Holmes–you all inspire me in so many ways, and I am incredibly grateful for your friendship over the years! Even when we don't see each other often, we always pick up right where we left off!

To everyone who preordered a copy of my book–OMG y'all have no freaking idea how much seeing your orders pop up in my inbox kept me pushing through...up until the very last minute of this massive project! Thank you for believing in me and being my early supporters!

To anyone who ever attended my fitness classes–in person or virtually–I hope you know how much your kind words kept me showing up to teach, even when I was feeling self-conscious.

To my lovely beauty crew for helping me to stay confident while taking big leaps of faith: Shannon Bashant for making my hair look good, Gwen and Sky at Ava Nail & Lash for giving my lashes life and keeping my nails glamorous!

Also, to the incredible women in business who helped me pull off this project–Alicia Ifill for the fabulous cover photo; Eve Aguilar for the beautiful cover designs; Mar Dolan for busting out some serious editing during the home stretch of this project; Dr. Moira Hanna for setting up the coworking calls through the Female Entrepreneur Association (FEA); Erin (Geib) Hamaoui for helping me bring the Melyssa with a WHY brand to life; Sarah Grey for being such a tech wizard and reviving my websites; Adela Novotna for creating my email campaign for this book launch; Monica Delgado for being such a strong cheerleader in my life and woman-owned business inspiration; Mari Milenkovic and the Her

Brand & Co. Team for helping me begin to create strategy among my multipassionate mess of a business; Alexa Cawley and The Friday Society members–I can't wait to start getting back on our calls together; to Kam Niskach, the MetKon Instructors, and the KPOW Krew–your positivity and consistency with your own well-being habits helped me stay focused on my own during this book writing process; Jenni-Lyn Williams for creating magical tea blends that helped me keep my sanity while writing this book (*seriously Jenni-Lyn, your Calm the F*ck Down tea kept me from a few good breakdowns during this whole writing journey!*); my Womantrepreneur crew for helping me to stay on track and commit to making this happen this year!

To all of my secret women in business mentors–Carrie Green, Denise Duffield-Thomas, Gina Devee, Jen Sincero, Mel Robbins, Lizzo–your words and actions continuously inspire me to believe in myself and give me hope for making my dream life a reality! To Amanda Frances for partnering with Cara Alwill to bring the course Self-Published to life and help me find the balls to actually follow through with this dream of writing my own book! And extra special thanks to my woman in business icon–Cara Alwill–you helped me to realize that I can be successful and embrace my authentic self. The freedom I have found from following your journey over the last few years, reading your books, and listening to your podcast was just the permission I needed to break out of the corporate chains and show up as my true self!

To Andy Grammer for this **phenomenal** music for basically being the soundtrack to my life–your songs *Damn It Feels Good to be Me, Love Myself,* and *The Wrong Party* were my jams for when I needed to reconnect with myself. The amount of healing that your words have given me over the years–I will never be able to fully explain it!

To the UCF Clinical Psychology Master's Program faculty–thank you for reminding me that empathy is a strength, self-care is a necessity, and allowing me the chance to pursue my passions.

To The UCF Recreation and Wellness Center staff–the lifelong friends that I have made from working as a lifeguard during undergrad to falling in love with fitness during graduate school. Special thanks to Valerie Reed for helping me sort through my life priorities when I was lost in the doctoral program, and thanks to Troy Morris for pushing me to obtain my personal training certification–even though I didn't think I was "cut out" for it.

To Dr. Diane Robinson, Nicole Santapola, and the entire Integrative Medicine team–you all helped me get better in tune with the mind-body connection and first introduced me to the field of lifestyle medicine. Thank you for helping me gain valuable clinical experience!

To the American College of Lifestyle Medicine for helping me find my tribe of like-minded people–I knew I wasn't out of my mind for trying to find the link between fitness and mental health and how I could turn it into a career!

To the Lake Nona Performance Club and Dr. Sharon Wasserstrom–thank you for including me on your inaugural Medical Advisory Council to help bring lifestyle medicine to the Lake Nona community.

To the people who tried their best to tell me I had to look or act a certain way to find success. Thank you for showing me what I didn't want out of my life–it gave me the courage to bet on myself.

To the people who have always believed in me, supported me, and cheered me on–*I love you all so much!*

To the animals that I have worked with over the years that humbled me many times and taught me soooo many lessons! The most important of those lessons–live in the moment, have fun, and don't care about what others think of you!

In Memoriam
—
To the people who were gone too soon in life...
My godparents – Auntie Linda & Uncle Marty
My dear friend, Bre the Braveheart
My wild Uncle Jerry

ABOUT MELYSSA

Melyssa Allen is a respected speaker, board-certified lifestyle medicine professional, and certified health and well-being coach dedicated to making healthy living fun and accessible through "edutainment" experiences. Melyssa founded her company, Melyssa with a WHY, LLC, to help individuals, companies, and communities adopt habits to support happier and healthier lifestyles. Using her multidisciplinary training in mental health counseling, wellness coaching, and lifestyle medicine with over a decade of behavior change experience, Melyssa is passionate about guiding people to build lasting, positive health habits.

Melyssa uses her strengths of Positivity, Humor, and Zest to captivate her audiences through speaking engagements, group fitness experiences, online courses, and coaching programs. She considers her approach a combination of sassy and scholarly and delivers a blend of both entertainment and education during her presentations.

Melyssa has served on the Medical Advisory Council at the Lake Nona Performance Club and as the Secretary for the ACLM Fitness in Medicine Member Interest Group.

Melyssa is a dedicated dog mom to her sweet Buddy-boy, and new cat mom to Jackie the kitty.

CONNECT WITH MELYSSA

Learn more about Melyssa at www.melyssawithawhy.com

Connect with Melyssa on social media at:
IG: @melyssa_with_a_why
LinkedIn: Melyssa Allen

To request additional information about Melyssa's speaking engagements, healthy living workshops, and well-being coaching services, send an email to info@melyssawithawhy.com

RECOMMENDED RESOURCES

ONLINE

- **Book Website:** https://healthylivingdoesnthavetosuck.com
- **Bonuses:** healthylivingdoesnthavetosuck.com/bonus
- **Melyssa with a WHY Company Website:** www.melyssawithawhy.com
- **Instagram Page:** @healthylivingdoesnthavetosuck
- **Change Maker Community:** https://www.facebook.com/groups/healthylivingdoesnthavetosuck
- **Insight Timer Meditation App:** https://insighttimer.com
- **American College of Lifestyle Medicine Website:** https://lifestylemedicine.org
- **Full Plate Living:** https://www.fullplateliving.org
- **American College of Sports Medicine (ACSM) Exercise is Medicine ®:** https://www.exerciseismedicine.org
- **American Academy of Sleep Medicine:** https://sleepeducation.org
- **Blue Zones:** https://www.bluezones.com/

BOOKS

- Ali, S. (2018). *The Self-Love Workbook: A Life-Changing Guide to Boost Self-Esteem, Recognize Your Worth and Find Genuine Happiness*. Simon and Schuster.
- Brewer, J. (2022). *Unwinding anxiety: New science shows how to break the cycles of worry and fear to heal your mind*. Penguin.
- Brewer, J. (2017). The Craving Mind. In *The Craving Mind*. Yale University Press.
- Clear, J. (2018). *Atomic habits: An easy & proven way to build good habits & break bad ones*. Penguin.

- Duhigg, C. (2012). *The power of habit: Why we do what we do in life and business* (Vol. 34, No. 10). Random House.
- Dweck, C. S. (2006). *Mindset: The new psychology of success.* Random House.
- Fogg, B. J. (2019). *Tiny habits: The small changes that change everything.* Eamon Dolan Books.
- Harris, R. (2011). *The confidence gap: A guide to overcoming fear and self-doubt.* Shambhala Publications.
- Harris, R. (2022). *The happiness trap: How to stop struggling and start living.* Shambhala Publications.
- Lianov, L. (2019). *Roots of Positive Change: Optimizing Health Care with Positive Psychology.* American College of Lifestyle Medicine.
- McGonigal, K. (2016). *The upside of stress: Why stress is good for you, and how to get good at it.* Penguin.
- McGonigal, K. (2019). *The Joy of Movement: How exercise helps us find happiness, hope, connection, and courage.* Penguin.
- Prochaska, J. O., & Prochaska, J. M. (2016). *Changing to thrive: using the stages of change to overcome the top threats to your health and happiness.* Simon and Schuster.
- Robbins, M. (2021). *The High 5 Habit: Take Control of Your Life with One Simple Habit.* Hay House, Inc.
- Robbins, M. (2017). *The 5 second rule: Transform your life, work, and confidence with everyday courage.* Simon and Schuster.
- Shapiro, S. (2020). *Good Morning, I Love You: Mindfulness and Self-compassion Practices to Rewire Your Brain for Calm, Clarity, and Joy.* Sounds True.

REFERENCES

Chapter 1: "You Are HERE!"

- Berkman, E. T. (2018). Value-based choice: An integrative, neuroscience-informed model of health goals. *Psychology & health, 33*(1), 40-57.
- Carden, L., & Wood, W. (2018). Habit formation and change. *Current opinion in behavioral sciences, 20,* 117-122.
- Ceceli, A. O., & Tricomi, E. (2018). Habits and goals: a motivational perspective on action control. *Current Opinion in Behavioral Sciences, 20,* 110-116.
- Kingston, K. M., & Hardy, L. (1997). Effects of different types of goals on processes that support performance. *The Sport Psychologist, 11*(3), 277-293.
- Kruglanski, A. W., & Szumowska, E. (2020). Habitual behavior is goal-driven. *Perspectives on Psychological Science, 15*(5), 1256-1271.
- Wood, W., & Neal, D. T. (2016). Healthy through habit: Interventions for initiating & maintaining health behavior change. *Behavioral Science & Policy, 2*(1), pp. 71–83.
- Zhang, C. Q., Leeming, E., Smith, P., Chung, P. K., Hagger, M. S., & Hayes, S. C. (2018). Acceptance and commitment therapy for health behavior change: a contextually-driven approach. *Frontiers in psychology,* 2350.

Chapter 2: Mindset Matters

- Beck, J. S. (2020). *Cognitive behavior therapy* (3rd ed.). Guilford Press.

- Brewer, J. A., Davis, J. H., & Goldstein, J. (2013). Why is it so hard to pay attention, or is it? Mindfulness, the factors of awakening and reward-based learning. *Mindfulness, 4*(1), 75-80.
- Harris, R. (2019). *ACT made simple: An easy-to-read primer on acceptance and commitment therapy.* New Harbinger Publications.
- Hayes, S. C. (2019). Acceptance and commitment therapy: towards a unified model of behavior change. *World psychiatry, 18*(2), 226.
- Shapiro, S. L., Carlson, L. E., Astin, J. A., & Freedman, B. (2006). Mechanisms of mindfulness. *Journal of clinical psychology, 62*(3), 373-386.
- Shapiro, S. L., Oman, D., Thoresen, C. E., Plante, T. G., & Flinders, T. (2008). Cultivating mindfulness: effects on well-being. *Journal of clinical psychology, 64*(7), 840-862.
- Wright, J. H., Brown, G. K., Thase, M. E., & Basco, M. R. (2017). *Learning cognitive-behavior therapy: An illustrated guide.* American Psychiatric Pub.

Chapter 3: Acceptance and Authenticity

- de Vries, D. A., Möller, A. M., Wieringa, M. S., Eigenraam, A. W., & Hamelink, K. (2018). Social comparison as the thief of joy: Emotional consequences of viewing strangers' Instagram posts. *Media psychology, 21*(2), 222-245.
- Jiang, S., & Ngien, A. (2020). The effects of Instagram use, social comparison, and self-esteem on social anxiety: A survey study in Singapore. *Social Media+ Society, 6*(2), 2056305120912488.
- Kleemans, M., Daalmans, S., Carbaat, I., & Anschütz, D. (2018). Picture perfect: The direct effect of manipulated Instagram photos on body image in adolescent girls. *Media Psychology, 21*(1), 93-110.

- Ota, C., & Nakano, T. (2021). Neural correlates of beauty retouching to enhance attractiveness of self-depictions in women. *Social Neuroscience, 16*(2), 121-133.

Chapter 4: Positive Health & Lifestyle Medicine

- *Authentic happiness.* University of Pennsylvania. (n.d.) from https://www.authentichappiness.sas.upenn.edu/learn/positivehea lth
- *CDC data show U.S. Life Expectancy continues to decline.* AAFP. (2018, December 10) from https://www.aafp.org/news/health-of-the-public/20181210lifeexpectdrop.html
- Centers for Disease Control and Prevention. (2022, August 31). *Life expectancy in the U.S. dropped for the second year in a row in 2021.* Centers for Disease Control and Prevention from https://www.cdc.gov/nchs/pressroom/nchs_press_releases/2022/20220831.htm
- Emmons, R. A., & McCullough, M. E. (2003). Counting blessings versus burdens: an experimental investigation of gratitude and subjective well-being in daily life. *Journal of personality and social psychology, 84*(2), 377.
- *Exploring the concept of Positive Health.* RWJF. (2020, February 12) from https://www.rwjf.org/en/library/research/2017/08/exploring-the-concept-of-positive-health.html
- Faries, M. D. (2016). Why we don't "just do it" understanding the intention-behavior gap in lifestyle medicine. *American journal of lifestyle medicine, 10*(5), 322-329.
- Frates, B. (2019). *Lifestyle medicine handbook: An introduction to the power of healthy habits.* Healthy Learning.
- Fredrickson, B. L., & Joiner, T. (2018). Reflections on positive emotions and upward spirals. *Perspectives on Psychological Science, 13*(2), 194-199.

- Garland, E. L., Fredrickson, B., Kring, A. M., Johnson, D. P., Meyer, P. S., & Penn, D. L. (2010). Upward spirals of positive emotions counter downward spirals of negativity: Insights from the broaden-and-build theory and affective neuroscience on the treatment of emotion dysfunctions and deficits in psychopathology. *Clinical psychology review, 30*(7), 849-864.
- Kashdan, T. B., & Ciarrochi, J. V. (Eds.). (2013). *Mindfulness, acceptance, and positive psychology: The seven foundations of well-being.* New Harbinger Publications.
- Kotifani, A. (n.d.). *Power 9®.* Blue Zones. Retrieved October 11, 2022, from https://www.bluezones.com/2016/11/power-9/
- Kreouzi, M., Theodorakis, N., & Constantinou, C. (2022). Lessons Learned From Blue Zones, Lifestyle Medicine Pillars and Beyond: An Update on the Contributions of Behavior and Genetics to Wellbeing and Longevity. *American Journal of Lifestyle Medicine,* 15598276221118494.
- Lianov, L. (2019). *Roots of Positive Change: Optimizing Health Care with Positive Psychology.* American College of Lifestyle Medicine.
- Lianov, L. S., Fredrickson, B. L., Barron, C., Krishnaswami, J., & Wallace, A. (2019). Positive psychology in lifestyle medicine and health care: strategies for implementation. *American journal of lifestyle medicine, 13*(5), 480-486.
- Louie, D., Brook, K., & Frates, E. (2016). The laughter prescription: a tool for lifestyle medicine. *American journal of lifestyle medicine, 10*(4), 262-267.
- Morton, D. P. (2018). Combining lifestyle medicine and positive psychology to improve mental health and emotional well-being. *American journal of lifestyle medicine, 12*(5), 370-374.
- Prochaska, J. J., & Prochaska, J. O. (2011). A review of multiple health behavior change interventions for primary prevention. *American journal of lifestyle medicine, 5*(3), 208-221.
- Rippe, J. M. (2018). Lifestyle medicine: the health promoting power of daily habits and practices. *American journal of lifestyle medicine, 12*(6), 499-512.

- *What is positive health?* positive. (n.d.) from
  https://positivehealthresearch.org/about

Chapter 5: Invest in Your Rest

- Barnes, C. M., & Drake, C. L. (2015). Prioritizing sleep health: public health policy recommendations. *Perspectives on Psychological Science, 10*(6), 733-737.
- Buysse, D. J. (2014). Sleep health: can we define it? Does it matter?. *Sleep, 37*(1), 9-17.
- Dedhia, P., & Maurer, R. (2022). Sleep and Health—A Lifestyle Medicine Approach. *Journal of Family Practice, 71*(1), S30-S30.
- Dzierzewski, J. M., Sabet, S. M., Ghose, S. M., Perez, E., Soto, P., Ravyts, S. G., & Dautovich, N. D. (2021). Lifestyle factors and sleep health across the lifespan. *International Journal of Environmental Research and Public Health, 18*(12), 6626.
- Gurley, V. F. (2019). Sleep as medicine and lifestyle medicine for optimal sleep. In *Lifestyle Medicine* (pp. 995-1001). CRC Press.
- Magnavita, N., & Garbarino, S. (2017). Sleep, health and wellness at work: a scoping review. *International journal of environmental research and public health, 14*(11), 1347.
- National Sleep Foundation.
- Van Straten, A., van der Zweerde, T., Kleiboer, A., Cuijpers, P., Morin, C. M., & Lancee, J. (2018). Cognitive and behavioral therapies in the treatment of insomnia: a meta-analysis. *Sleep medicine reviews, 38*, 3-16.

Chapter 6: Stress Less

- Baban, K. A., & Morton, D. P. (2022). Lifestyle Medicine and Stress Management. *The Journal of Family Practice, 71*(1 Suppl Lifestyle), S24-S29.

- Braun, C., Foreyt, J. P., & Johnston, C. A. (2016). Stress: a core lifestyle issue. *American journal of lifestyle medicine, 10*(4), 235-238.
- McGonigal, K. (2013). How to make stress your friend. *Ted Global, Edinburgh, Scotland, 6*, 13.
- Merlo, G., & Vela, A. (2022). Mental health in lifestyle medicine: A call to action. *American Journal of Lifestyle Medicine, 16*(1), 7-20.
- Phillips, E. M., Frates, E. P., & Park, D. J. (2020). Lifestyle medicine. *Physical Medicine and Rehabilitation Clinics, 31*(4), 515-526.

Chapter 7: Choose Less Booze

- *Alcohol and cancer risk fact sheet*. National Cancer Institute. (n.d.) from https://www.cancer.gov/about-cancer/causes-prevention/risk/alcohol/alcohol-fact-sheet
- *Breast cancer risk: Drinking alcohol*. Susan G. Komen®. (2022, October 3) from https://www.komen.org/breast-cancer/risk-factor/alcohol-consumption/
- Centers for Disease Control and Prevention. (2022, April 19). *Facts about moderate drinking*. Centers for Disease Control and Prevention. from https://www.cdc.gov/alcohol/fact-sheets/moderate-drinking.htm
- Daviet, R., Aydogan, G., Jagannathan, K., Spilka, N., Koellinger, P. D., Kranzler, H. R., ... & Wetherill, R. R. (2022). Associations between alcohol consumption and gray and white matter volumes in the UK Biobank. Nature communications, 13(1), 1-11.
- Hamajima N, Hirose K, Tajima K, et al. for the Collaborative Group on Hormonal Factors in Breast Cancer. Alcohol, tobacco and breast cancer—collaborative reanalysis of individual data from 53 epidemiological studies, including 58,515 women with breast cancer and 95,067 women without the disease. Br J Cancer. 87(11):1234-45, 2002.

- *Health effects*. smokefree gov. (n.d.) from https://smokefree.gov/quit-smoking/why-you-should-quit/health-effects
- Rock CL, Thomson C, Gansler T, et al. American Cancer Society guideline for diet and physical activity for cancer prevention. CA Cancer J Clin. 70(4):245-271, 2020.
- U.S. Department of Health and Human Services. (n.d.). *Rethinking drinking homepage - NIAAA*. National Institute on Alcohol Abuse and Alcoholism from https://www.rethinkingdrinking.niaaa.nih.gov/
- Zahr, N. M., Kaufman, K. L., & Harper, C. G. (2011). Clinical and pathological features of alcohol-related brain damage. *Nature Reviews Neurology, 7*(5), 284-294.

Chapter 8: Let's Move

- Islam H, Gibala MJ, Little JP. Exercise Snacks: A Novel Strategy to Improve Cardiometabolic Health. Exerc Sport Sci Rev. 2022 Jan 1;50(1):31-37. doi: 10.1249/JES.0000000000000275.
- Lobelo, F., Stoutenberg, M., & Hutber, A. (2014). The exercise is medicine global health initiative: a 2014 update. *British journal of sports medicine, 48*(22), 1627-1633.
- Otto, M., & Smits, J. A. (2011). *Exercise for mood and anxiety: Proven strategies for overcoming depression and enhancing well-being*. OUP USA.
- Pedersen, B. K., & Saltin, B. (2015). Exercise as medicine–evidence for prescribing exercise as therapy in 26 different chronic diseases. *Scandinavian journal of medicine & science in sports, 25*, 1-72.
- Rep, M. M. M. W. (2004). ACSM's Exercise Is Medicine™: A Clinician's Guide to Exercise Prescription. *Prev Med, 39*, 815-822.

Chapter 9: Good Mood Food

- American College of Lifestyle Medicine (ACLM) Food as Medicine Jumpstart. *Patient resources.* American College of Lifestyle Medicine. (2022, October 25) from https://lifestylemedicine.org/project/patient-resources/
- Blanchflower DG, Oswald AJ, Stewart- Brown S. Is psychological well-being linked to the consumption of fruit and vegetables? *Soc Indic Res.* 2013;114:785-801.
- Brewer, J. A., Ruf, A., Beccia, A. L., Essien, G. I., Finn, L. M., Lutterveld, R. V., & Mason, A. E. (2018). Can mindfulness address maladaptive eating behaviors? Why traditional diet plans fail and how new mechanistic insights may lead to novel interventions. *Frontiers in Psychology*, 1418.
- *Full plate living - A doable approach to healthy living.* Full Plate Living - A doable approach to healthy living. (n.d.). from https://www.fullplateliving.org/
- Naidoo, U. (2021). Eat to Beat Stress. *American Journal of Lifestyle Medicine, 15*(1), 39-42.
- NCI Staff. (2021, July 22). *Red Meat Genetic signature for colorectal cancer.* National Cancer Institute from https://www.cancer.gov/news-events/cancer-currents-blog/2021/red-meat-colorectal-cancer-genetic-signature
- *The health at every size® (HAES®) principles.* ASDAH. (2022, April 22). Retrieved November 4, 2022, from https://asdah.org/health-at-every-size-haes-approach/

Chapter 10: Stop Slips from Becoming Slides

- Abascal, L., Vela, A., Sugden, S., Kohlenberg, S., Hirschberg, A., Young, A., ... & Merlo, G. (2022). Incorporating Mental Health Into Lifestyle Medicine. *American Journal of Lifestyle Medicine*, 15598276221084250.

- Baska, A., Kurpas, D., Kenkre, J., Vidal-Aaball, J., Petrazzuoli, F., Dolan, M., ... & Robins, J. (2021). Social prescribing and lifestyle medicine—a remedy to chronic health problems?. *International Journal of Environmental Research and Public Health, 18*(19), 10096.
- Duncan, A. R., Jaini, P. A., & Hellman, C. M. (2021). Positive psychology and hope as lifestyle medicine modalities in the therapeutic encounter: a narrative review. *American Journal of Lifestyle Medicine, 15*(1), 6-13.
- Franklin, N. C., & Tate, C. A. (2009). Lifestyle and successful aging: An overview. *American Journal of Lifestyle Medicine, 3*(1), 6-11.
- Moniz-Lewis, D. I., Stein, E. R., Bowen, S., & Witkiewitz, K. (2022). Self-Efficacy as a Potential Mechanism of Behavior Change in Mindfulness-Based Relapse Prevention. *Mindfulness, 13*(9), 2175-2185.
- Pathak, N., & Pollard, K. J. (2021). Lifestyle medicine prescriptions for personal and planetary health. *The Journal of Climate Change and Health, 4*, 100077.
- Raypole, C. (2020, June 17). *Hugging self: Benefits, how to do it, and more.* Healthline from https://www.healthline.com/health/hugging-self#more-self-love
- Schwarzer, R. (2008). Modeling health behavior change: How to predict and modify the adoption and maintenance of health behaviors. *Applied psychology, 57*(1), 1-29.
- Zimmerman, R. S., & Connor, C. (1989). Health promotion in context: The effects of significant others on health behavior change. *Health Education Quarterly, 16*(1), 57-75.

Chapter 11: Your ACTION Plan

- Gardner, B., & Rebar, A. L. (2019). Habit formation and behavior change. In *Oxford research encyclopedia of psychology.*

- Prochaska, J. J., Spring, B., & Nigg, C. R. (2008). Multiple health behavior change research: an introduction and overview. *Preventive medicine, 46*(3), 181-188.
- Noar, S. M., Chabot, M., & Zimmerman, R. S. (2008). Applying health behavior theory to multiple behavior change: considerations and approaches. *Preventive medicine, 46*(3), 275-280.